A Prominent Professor's Interpretation of Huangdi's Inner Canon of Medicine
The Five Zang-Organs

名师解读黄帝内经·五脏篇

翟双庆 **著**

吴 青 李晓莉 **主译**

陈铸芬 刘艾娟 石 径 谢文鑫 周阿剑 **译**

中国海洋大学出版社

· 青岛 ·

图书在版编目（CIP）数据

名师解读黄帝内经．五脏篇／翟双庆著；吴青，李
晓莉主译．-- 青岛：中国海洋大学出版社，2023.5（2023.11重印）

ISBN 978-7-5670-3399-3

Ⅰ．①名…　Ⅱ．①翟…②吴…③李…　Ⅲ．①《内经
》－五脏－养生（中医）　Ⅳ．① R221 ② R223.1

中国国家版本馆 CIP 数据核字（2023）第 043573 号

出版发行	中国海洋大学出版社
社　　址	青岛市香港东路 23 号　　　　邮政编码　266071
出 版 人	刘文菁
网　　址	http://pub.ouc.edu.cn
订购电话	0532－82032573（传真）
责任编辑	付绍瑜　　　　　　　　电　　话　0532－85902533
印　　制	日照日报印务中心
版　　次	2023 年 5 月第 1 版
印　　次	2023 年 11 月第 2 次印刷
成品尺寸	170 mm×240 mm
印　　张	14.75
字　　数	272 千
印　　数	1001～1800
定　　价	60.00 元

发现印装质量问题，请致电 18663037500，由印刷厂负责调换。

· Foreword by Prof. Fang Tingyu ·

Traditional Chinese Medicine (TCM) is regarded as one of the representative symbols of Chinese culture. With its emphasis on a holistic view, maintaining balance of *yin* and *yang*, and nurturing life to enjoy health and longevity, it has gained increasing recognition and wider acceptance amongst people in and outside China. According to China's National Administration of Traditional Chinese Medicine (NATCM), as of October 2020, TCM has spread to 196 countries and regions. It has been found to be effective not only in global defense against malaria, but also in guarding against COVID-19.

What is TCM? What are the medical beliefs of the Chinese people? What is the cause of disease? What are the basic principles and strategies of TCM treatment? How should we stay healthy? The answers to these questions can be found in *Huangdi's Inner Canon of Medicine* (*Huáng Dì Nèi Jīng* 黄帝内经), which is considered to be the most influential medical classic in existence and has therefore been accorded first place among medical works in China. The book contains two parts: *Fundamental Questions* (*Sù Wèn* 素问) and *Miraculous Pivot* (*Líng Shū* 灵枢). The former mainly explains the basic TCM theories, whereas the latter elaborates on the art of acupuncture.

Huangdi's Inner Canon of Medicine tops the reading list for university TCM students and for those who hope to gain access to TCM. As it was compiled in the Western Han dynasty (206 BC–AD 25), the text was written in classical Chinese without any punctuation, which brings considerable language difficulties to present-day Chinese and Western readers.

To assist the general public in understanding the book, scholars have been working hard to offer vernacular Chinese, annotations, analyses, and commentaries upon the text. Among them, a series of books authored by Prof. Zhai Shuangqing (翟双庆) are part of the best efforts. They include the topics of the five *zang*-organs, six *qi*, seven emotions, longevity, and diagnosis and treatment.

Before the whole text of *Huangdi's Inner Canon of Medicine* was translated into English, some short passages of the book had been translated into Western languages. In 1949, Ilza Veith published her English version, which contains Chapters 1–34 in *Fundamental Questions* along with a 76–page research text. As of July 2022, a total of 24 English versions of the book have been published by Chinese and foreign scholars. While all versions are targeted to readers who are eager to immerse themselves in the profundity of TCM theory, how the majority of lay people in Western countries can gain access to TCM theory remains to be explored.

In the times of bio-psycho-social medicine, a more holistic and comprehensive medical model is required. TCM emphasizes the correspondence between man and nature as well as the maintenance of physical, mental, and spiritual balance alongside social wellness. It prioritizes disease prevention. In English-speaking countries, people believe that an apple a day keeps a doctor away. In China, there are a number of adages informing people of the right things to do to keep fit or to prevent disease. For example, diligence cultivates skills while laziness invites malady; aged *Aiye* (Argy Wormwood Leaf) at home keeps healers away; and smiles make one look younger. These words of wisdom contribute to the health and longevity of those who know the right way to keep fit. An English book that contains such Chinese wisdom and medical philosophy is believed to bring benefits to a wider reading circle.

A Prominent Professor's Interpretation of Huangdi's Inner Canon of Medicine: The Five Zang-Organs is a translated version based on the renowned work by Prof. Zhai Shuangqing, i.e., *Zhai Shuang Qing Jie Du Huang Di Nei Jing Wu Zang Pian* (翟双庆解读黄帝内经·五脏篇). It is the first of his series of books in Chinese. The book gives an overview of the five *zang*-organs, i.e., heart, liver, spleen, lung, and kidney, and identifies the conceptual difference between TCM and modern medicine. Furthermore, it illustrates the functions and disorders of related *zang*-organs. Particularly, it tells us how to prevent disorder and nurture health. The author explains the profound TCM theory in simple language with annotations, medical cases, and stories from Chinese literary classics, making it an appropriate starting point for those who desire to gain an understanding into *Huangdi's Inner Canon of Medicine*.

In the process of translation, the translators have made every effort to render the text easy to read. They changed the monologic writing format of the original into a question-and-answer format so that the readers are able to quickly identify the main ideas. Coincidently, it matches the writing style of *Huangdi's Inner Canon of Medicine*, in which it takes the form of dialogues between Huangdi and his ministers such as Qibo and Bogao. In addition, various means such as *pinyin*, Chinese characters, notes, tables, figures, or examples are used where necessary to facilitate readers' understanding. The tone of some statements was softened to bridge the cultural gap and things that may induce misunderstanding were removed. In this sense, the book can be a feasible research subject for those who are interested in TCM translation studies.

All roads lead to Rome. This book in your hand is an interesting and inspirational attempt to tell TCM stories in plain language. It is hoped that readers at home and abroad would enjoy reading it, and get a glimpse of how TCM understands the human body and its vital organs.

Fang Tingyu
Beijing University of Chinese Medicine
Summer, 2022

· Foreword ·

Huangdi's Inner Canon of Medicine (*Huáng Dì Nèi Jīng* 黄帝内经 , or the *Canon*) is the earliest extant medical classic in China. It is one of the two ancient Chinese medical books listed on the Memory of the World Register and has played an indelible role in the inheritance and development of Traditional Chinese Medicine (TCM). To help the lay people understand the classic and promote awareness of health preservation, Prof. Zhai Shuangqing (翟双庆) of Beijing University of Chinese Medicine, Chairman of Nei Jing Branch of the China Association of Chinese Medicine, was invited to give a series of lectures on *Huangdi's Inner Canon of Medicine* on China Central Television (CCTV) Channel 10 'Lecture Room' program. Different from his university lectures, Prof. Zhai adopted a thematic approach to retell the story by analyzing the main ideas of *Huangdi's Inner Canon of Medicine* according to such topics as the five *zang*-organs, six *qi*, seven emotions, longevity, as well as diagnosis and treatment. Making use of his over 30 years of research experience and profound understanding of the theories in *Huangdi's Inner Canon of Medicine*, Prof. Zhai interpreted the classic in an accessible manner. He decoded Chinese characters, included in his presentations citations of ancient Chinese classics, and incorporated legends, stories and medical cases by the distinguished physicians. The TV program was so well-received that each of his seminars was transcribed and compiled into a series of books published by the Science Publishing Press (2016, 2017 and 2018), People's Medical Publishing House (2020), and

China Press of Traditional Chinese Medicine (2020, 2021). In 2023, the series were awarded '2022 Top 100 National Excellent Popular Science Works' by the Ministry of Science and Technology of the People's Republic of China.

This book was adapted and translated from the first part of the TV series: *Zhai Shuangqing's Interpretation of Huangdi's Inner Canon of Medicine: The Five Zang-Organs (Zhái Shuāng Qìng Jiě Dú Huáng Dì Nèi Jīng Wǔ Zàng Piān* 翟双庆解读黄帝内经•五脏篇). It focuses on the five *zang*-organs i.e., heart, liver, spleen, lung[①], and kidney, as they are fitting embodiments of the ancient Chinese way of thinking— *yin* and *yang*, the five elements or phases, image thinking (*xiàng sī wéi* 象思维) as well as the essence-*qi* theory to understand the human body. Understanding the five *zang*-organs can help people understand themselves and their body. This is of great significance for healthcare and disease prevention.

To better present the key points from the original version, we rearranged the contents of each chapter in a question-and-answer format and translated it with reference to some of Prof. Zhai's lecture notes for his massive open online course (MOOC). In addition, we added some Chinese *pinyin* and their equivalent characters, a dynasty's time period, tables, illustrations, and notes where necessary to facilitate understanding and avoid misinterpretation. Prof. Wu Qing managed the translation project and translated Chapters 1–5 and Chapter 12. Prof. Wu also provided quality assurance and improved the entire 17 chapters of the translated version. Li Xiaoli and Xie Wenxin translated Chapters 6–7 and helped with proofreading. Liu Aijuan translated Chapters 8–9; Chen Zhufen translated Chapters 10–11; Zhou Ajian translated Chapters 13–14; and Shi Jing translated Chapters 15–17.

The key reference books used in the translation of some TCM terms and quotations included the following:

Li, Zhaoguo. *Yellow Emperor's Canon of Medicine · Plain Conversation*[M]. Beijing: World Publishing Corporation, 2005.

Unschuld, Paul and Tessenow, Hermann in collaboration with Zheng, Jinsheng. *Huang Di Nei Jing Su Wen: An Annotated Translation of Huang Di's Inner Classic – Basic Questions*[M]. Berkeley: University of California Press, 2011.

---

① lung: used in singular form to refer to the concept in TCM, which is different from that in biomedicine. So is the kidney.

Unschuld, Paul. *Huang Di Nei Jing Ling Shu: The Ancient Classic on Needle Therapy*[M]. Berkeley: University of California Press, 2016.

Xie, Zhufan and Xie, Fang. 2019. *Classified Dictionary of Traditional Chinese Medicine* [M]. 2nd new edition. Beijing: Foreign Languages Press, 2019.

Chapter 1 gives a brief introduction to *Huangdi's Inner Canon of Medicine* including its content, authorship, completion time, transmission, the meaning of the titles, the embedded thoughts, and the way of thinking; Chapters 2–5 deal with the heart (known as monarch); Chapters 6–9, the liver (known as general); Chapters 10–12, the spleen and the stomach (known as granary officer); Chapters 13–14, the lung (known as prime minister); and Chapters 15–17, the kidney (known as labor officer).

TCM is a medical system different from biomedicine. It is not just a doctrine and a medical art, but more of a culture. Reading and understanding *Huangdi's Inner Canon of Medicine* is one of the exciting ways to approach Chinese health culture. As Prof. Zhai Shuangqing says, by introducing the five *zang*-organs based on *Huangdi's Inner Canon of Medicine*, we not only offer an insight into this classical medical work, into TCM and traditional Chinese culture, but also provide a different perspective for people to understand the human body. We hope that readers can use the TCM knowledge and experience documented in this unique medical classic to preserve their health in a better way.

It is our sincere hope that this book can be a helpful resource to those who are willing to attend to their health, keen on learning TCM, and enthusiastic about incorporating TCM into other cultures in the world. Besides, it can be an aid to college or university students and teachers who are interested in disseminating TCM culture.

Wu Qing

Beijing University of Chinese Medicine

November 23, 2021

· **Preface** ·
(Chinese Edition, 2016)

The Chinese President Xi Jinping (习近平) stated: 'Traditional Chinese Medicine (TCM) is the treasure of ancient Chinese science and the key to the treasure house of Chinese civilization.' Being an essential part of traditional Chinese culture, TCM, especially its development, is an important way to realize the Chinese Dream. Its thousands of years of history indicates that its development follows the law of classical inheritance. To develop TCM, inherit traditional Chinese culture and realize the Chinese Dream, it is more than necessary to emphasize the studies on classics, especially TCM classics. Those who are learning TCM, who want to be great doctors, and who want to grasp and inherit the essence of traditional Chinese culture must study and research TCM classics. Therefore, recent years have seen substantial popularization and publicity of TCM knowledge and classics on TV and Internet, in newspapers and other media.

Huangdi's Inner Canon of Medicine, or the *Canon*, was compiled in the Western Han dynasty (206 BC–AD 25) with a history of over two thousand years. Its publication marked the birth of TCM and the establishment of its theoretical system. With its unique theoretical thinking method, *Huangdi's Inner Canon of Medicine* has created the distinctive school of TCM in the world. It has played an irreplaceable role in the survival and prosperity of the Chinese nation and is still the escort of human health up to today. The book is known as the 'First Classic of TCM,' 'Ancient Encyclopedia,' 'Fascinating Writings Through the Ages,' and honored as 'The

Ancestral Art of Healers.' It is still desirable to explore the classic so that it serves humankind better. It adds the following values: to help people understand and make good use of the *Canon*; to form a healthy lifestyle; to develop self-management skills of disease prevention and healthcare; to employ the ideas and thoughts from the *Canon* for team building and collaboration. Its way of thinking can also be applied to the relationships of humankind with our ecosystem of nature, environment, society, and other aspects. This will ensure the Chinese communities increasingly cohesive. The *Canon* will play a more significant role in the process of realizing the great rejuvenation of the Chinese nation. To achieve this goal, the greatest priority is to make this classic accessible to the general public in China. Recently, we have published a series of popular science books related to *Huangdi's Inner Canon of Medicine* and held the first national contest on the knowledge contained in the book. We are now holding a relevant national essay contest entitled 'Read TCM Classics and Serve Healthy China.' All these are part of the popularization efforts.

In December 2015, Tu Youyou (屠呦呦) won the Nobel Prize for her discovery of artemisinin, an effective therapy for treating malaria. It is the first time a Chinese scientist has been awarded this honor. It has strengthened people's awareness that TCM is a great treasure house with great value. The year of 2016 marks the 60th anniversary of higher education in TCM. In China, the 60th year is a time for celebration, marking the beginning of the next circle of life. Now China has issued the Outline of the Strategic Plan on the Development of Traditional Chinese Medicine (2016-2030)[①]. Presently, it is the springtime for the development of TCM. On this occasion, I joined the well-regarded 'Lecture Room' program of CCTV Channel 10 and introduced *Huangdi's Inner Canon of Medicine* in a simple and accessible manner with medical cases and stories close to everyday life. I focused on traditional Chinese culture and explained its method of thinking while offering my own understanding of the classic. All the materials have been collated in this book to allow for enjoyable reading. It is my sincere hope that more people can have a better understanding of TCM including *Huangdi's Inner Canon of Medicine*, and make conscious use of its canonical wisdom. Any comments or suggestions will be

---

① Full text is availabe at www.gov.cn, retrieved on March 1, 2022.

appreciated.

Finally, I would like to extend my sincere gratitude to CCTV, the Science Publishing Press, and my students for their assistance with the video recording of the program and the compiling of this book.

Zhai Shuangqing

Beijing

March 28, 2016

· Acknowledgements ·

I acknowledge with immense gratitude the unyielding support and trust from Mr. Lin Jianping (林建平), Director of the Third Affiliated Hospital of Beijing University of Chinese Medicine (BUCM) and the former Director of the School of Humanities of BUCM where I have been teaching English. Without his motivation and constant encouragement, I would not have achieved what I have achieved in my career. It was indeed his initial hope that my colleagues and I could translate this book to disseminate Traditional Chinese Medicine and improve our expertise as well. This book would not have been completed without his urging and liaison. My thanks also go to Mr. Shao Chengjun (邵成军), Director of the Editorial Department of China Ocean University Press, for his interest and devoted efforts in having this book published. The publication of this book is funded by BUCM Research Grants (Grant No. 2020-JYB-ZDGG-091). Last but not the least, I am particularly indebted to Ying Chen for her untiring support and proof reading of the entire text.

Wu Qing

Beijing

November 23, 2021

· Contents ·

Chapter 1 The Mysterious *Canon* ···1

Chapter 2 The Monarch-like Heart ·······································15

Chapter 3 The Miraculous Heart Spirit·································23

Chapter 4 The Key to Emotional Regulation·······················34

Chapter 5 The Secret to Heart Fire ·····································48

Chapter 6 General's Power ··62

Chapter 7 General's Likes and Dislikes·······························72

Chapter 8 Causes of Fatigue ···82

Chapter 9 The Connection Between the Liver and Mood ·······95

Chapter 10 Granary Officer: The Spleen ·····························108

Chapter 11 Magic Functions of the Spleen and Stomach ········121

Chapter 12 Health Preservation of the Spleen and Stomach ······133

Chapter 13 Prime Minister: The Lung ································147

Chapter 14 The Delicate Lung ··160

Chapter 15 The Root of Prenatal Constitution: The Kidney·······172

Chapter 16 The Kidney's Miraculous Effects ······················183

Chapter 17 Nourishing the Kidney Is Nourishing Life·······193

Appendix Ⅰ Ancient Books ·······203

Appendix Ⅱ Some Chapters in *Huangdi's Inner Canon of Medicine*·······206

Appendix Ⅲ Chinese Medicinals·······211

Appendix Ⅳ Traditional Chinese Medicine Formulas·······214

Appendix Ⅴ Chronology of Chinese History·······216

Chapter 1
The Mysterious *Canon*

Q1. What is *Huangdi's Inner Canon of Medicine* (*Huáng Dì Nèi Jīng* 黄帝内经) about?

Huangdi's Inner Canon of Medicine is also known as *Yellow Emperor's Inner Canon of Medicine* or as *Inner Canon*. It is a medical classic, the first book on Traditional Chinese Medicine (TCM). There are two parts in the book: *Fundamental Questions* (*Sù Wèn* 素问) and *Miraculous Pivot* (*Líng Shū* 灵枢), each containing 81 chapters, amounting to a total of 162 chapters. Part 1 focuses on the fundamentals and theories of TCM and Part 2 on acupuncture therapies, i.e., acupoints and needles. *Fundamental Questions* includes Chinese ancestors' understanding on philosophy, astronomy, meteorology, geography, agriculture, and sociology. Sometimes, it is regarded as a book on other subjects rather than a medical book. For example, *History of Chinese Philosophy* (*Zhōng Guó Zhé Xué* 中国哲学) contains a chapter about it as a book on the ancient Chinese philosophy.

The theoretical part is the highlight. It includes the theory of *yin* and *yang*, the theory of five elements (*wǔ xíng* 五行), the theory of visceral manifestations (*zàng xiàng* 藏象), and the theory of *qi*, blood, essence (*jīng* 精), fluid (*yè* 液) and spirit (*shén* 神), offering insights into the human body that are different from biomedicine.

Interestingly, the book was written in the form of questions and answers, mostly between Huangdi and his ministers individually, including Qibo (岐伯)[①], Shaoshi (少师)[②] and Bogao (伯高)[③].

Huangdi's Inner Canon of Medicine is believed to be the earliest and the most important monograph on TCM. In 2011, it was listed in the Memory of the World Register along with *Compendium of Materia Medica* (*Běn Cǎo Gāng Mù* 本草纲目), another TCM masterpiece authored by Li Shizhen (李时珍) of the Ming dynasty (1368-1644).

Q2. Who wrote the book?

The authorship is not clearly recorded in the catalogue of ancient Chinese books. Some medical scholars believe that Huangdi is the author as the title suggests. Who is Huangdi, or Yellow Emperor? According to 'Records of the Historian: Annals of the Five Emperors' (*Shǐ Jì: Wǔ Dì Běn Jì* 史记•五帝本纪) and the opening chapter of *Huangdi's Inner Canon of Medicine*, 'In ancient times Huangdi was endowed with divine talents; while yet in early infancy he could speak; while still very young he was quick in comprehension; when he grew up he was sincere and wise; when he matured he ascended to the throne.' In fact, Huangdi was not a particular individual, but referred to a clan at the end of Chinese primitive society. It was a legend that Huangdi united the clans, taught people how to plant and sow, invented the south-pointing chariot, made boats, carriages, bows and arrows, cast musical instruments, developed medicine, and domesticated animals, which brought great benefits to people. It is simply because Huangdi had such a great influence on the development of the Chinese nation that the book was entitled *Huangdi's Inner Canon of Medicine* to imply its importance and authority. Liu An (刘安) of the Western Han dynasty stated in *Huainanzi* (*Huái Nán Zǐ* 淮南子): 'Because ancient people tended to command more respect than their contemporary fellows, it was

---

[①] Qibo (岐伯): a mythological Chinese doctor specialized in medicine and pulse theory.

[②] Shaoshi (少师): a mythological Chinese doctor specialized in body constitution.

[③] Bogao (伯高): a mythological Chinese doctor specialized in meridian theory.

common for Daoists to entrust their sayings to the ancestors such as Shennong (神农)① or Huangdi so that they could preach what they believed in an easy manner.' In ancient times, pseudonyms were considered stylish. By claiming it was Shennong's or Huangdi's book, it appeared self-evident that what was said held true. Several ancient Chinese books contain Shennong or Huangdi in their names, for instance, *Shennong's Herbal* (*Shén Nóng Běn Cǎo Jīng* 神农本草经), *Huangdi's Brightness Hall Classic* (*Huáng Dì Míng Táng Jīng* 黄帝明堂经) and *Huangdi's Eighty-one Difficult Issues* (*Huáng Dì Bā Shí Yī Nàn Jīng* 黄帝八十一难经). Consequently, the author Huangdi is a pseudonym. The inclusion of Huangdi in the title is due to the preference for antiquity, to enhance power of persuasion and attain recognition of the readers nationwide. A closer look would reveal that *Huangdi's Inner Canon of Medicine* is not a product from a single person in a single period because not all existent 162 chapters in the book share the same type of ideology. The style and rhetoric also vary from one text to another. It is thus very likely that the book is a collection of discourses by different authors at different times, more like conference proceedings of present-day academic practice.

Q3. When was the book completed?

The current edition of *Fundamental Questions* was compiled and put in order by Wang Bing (王冰) of the Tang dynasty (618–907) and the current edition of *Miraculous Pivot* was compiled by Shi Song (史崧) of the Southern Song dynasty (1127–1279). Nevertheless, neither bears the sign of its earlier version. Hence, the exact time of its earliest completed version has been heatedly debated throughout the history. To sum up, there are three main views: in the period of Huangdi, during the Spring and Autumn Period and the Warring States Period (770–221 BC) or in the Qin and Han dynasties (221 BC–AD 220).

The time of a book's completion refers to the time or era in which those scattered pages were put together in the form of a book. It is inappropriate to take

---

① Shengnong (神农): a mythological Chinese figure who invented agriculture and medicine and is well-known for the tale of Shennong tasting a hundred of herbs.

the time of emergence of an academic thought for the completion time of a book. Besides, a title should be given to the book. In other words, a book comes into being when bearing a title of its own, that is, the earliest record in literature. According to the above two criteria, the earliest extant record of *Huangdi's Inner Canon of Medicine* was found in 'The History of the Han Dynasty: Record on Art and Literature' (*Hàn Shū: Yì Wén Zhì* 汉书·艺文志) compiled by Ban Gu (班固), a Chinese historian, politician, and poet in the Eastern Han dynasty (25-220). Ban Gu cited it from *Seven Summaries* (*Qī Lüè* 七略) written by Liu Xiang (刘向, deceased 6 BC) and Liu Xin (刘歆, deceased AD 23) whose original version was lost but was fortunately collected in 'The History of the Han Dynasty: Record on Art and Literature'. The directory of *Seven Summaries* was compiled by Li Zhuguo (李柱国), a physician from a family that had practiced TCM for generations. Li lived in 26 BC in the Western Han dynasty, during the reign of Han Chengdi (汉成帝, reigned 32-7 BC). Research indicates that it is in 26 BC that he completed the directory of *Seven Summaries*. It is thus made clear that *Huangdi's Inner Canon of Medicine* was completed no later than 26 BC in the late period of the Western Han dynasty. At that time, the title of *Huangdi's Inner Canon of Medicine* was found in use.

A great deal of literature can be traced and referenced regarding the earliest possible time for completing *Huangdi's Inner Canon of Medicine*. It was not found available in such classics as *Master Lü's Spring and Autumn Annals* (*Lǚ Shì Chūn Qiū* 吕氏春秋), *Hanfeizi* (*Hán Fēi Zǐ* 韩非子) or *Luxuriant Gems of the Spring and Autumn Annals* (*Chūn Qiū Fán Lù* 春秋繁露), suggesting that *Huangdi's Inner Canon of Medicine* was not completed then. *Master Lü's Spring and Autumn Annals* was claimed to be an excellent book of its time owing to its inclusion of various schools of thought. It was so perfectly compiled that no fault was to be found— anyone who could spot an error in it would be rewarded a thousand pieces of gold. Even such a great book had no mention of *Huangdi's Inner Canon of Medicine*, which supported the idea that the *Canon* was not completed when *Master Lü's Spring and Autumn Annals* came to being.

Researchers also refer to another book—*Records of the Historian* (*Shǐ Jì* 史记), a landmark book written by Sima Qian (司马迁) who was a historian during the reign of Han Wudi (汉武帝, reigned 141–87 BC). It records a history of thousands of years and is sometimes regarded as an official monograph because its author Sima Qian was an official in charge of historical records. The book contains medical scripts including the biographies of doctors. Among them *Biographies of Bianque and Others* (*Biǎn Què Cāng Gōng Liè Zhuàn* 扁鹊仓公列传) is a special volume containing the biographies of many physicians and numerous other medical books, but no trace has been found of *Huangdi's Inner Canon of Medicine*. Therefore, *Huangdi's Inner Canon of Medicine* was not completed until *Records of the Historian* was written in 99 BC, the year that is generally believed to be when Sima Qian was imprisoned.

To conclude, the earliest time for the completion of *Huangdi's Inner Canon of Medicine* could be the same as that of *Records of the Historian*. To be specific, it was in between 99 BC and 26 BC that the compilation of the *Canon* was finished. Of course, the writing time of each of the 162 discourses would not be the same as the time when the entire book was compiled. Some may have come out earlier, others perhaps later. It is, therefore, not expected to determine the completion time of the book according to the specific time when a particular discourse is finished. Today, most scholars tend to believe that the compilation and publication of the *Canon* was accomplished in the mid and late periods of the Western Han Dynasty, after *Records of the Historian* and before *Seven Summaries*.

Q4. What do the titles mean?

Huangdi is a pseudonym, likely used to lend authority to the book. Then what does *Nei Jing* (内经) mean? According to 'History of the Han Dynasty: Record on Art and Literature,' there were seven medical classics available, i.e., *Huangdi's Inner Canon of Medicine, Huangdi's Outer Canon of Medicine* (*Huáng Dì Wài Jīng* 黄帝外经), *Bianque's Inner Classic* (*Biǎn Què Nèi Jīng* 扁鹊内经), *Bianque's Outer Classic* (*Biǎn Què Wài Jīng* 扁鹊外经), *Master Bai's Inner Classic* (*Bái Shì Nèi Jīng* 白氏内经), *Master Bai's Outer Classic* (*Bái Shì Wài Jīng* 白氏外经) and *Appended Chapters* (*Páng Piān* 旁篇). Of the seven classics, *Huangdi's Inner Canon of Medicine* is the only one that has been passed down to people today. *Huangdi's*

Inner Canon of Medicine is presumed to mainly expound the TCM theories whereas *Huangdi's Outer Canon of Medicine* primarily discusses treatment. The two books are seemingly related because of the literal words *nei* (inner) and *wai* (outer) in their titles. Some people, nevertheless, claim that no special meaning is attached to 'inner' or 'outer': they could simply refer to the first and the second parts of a book. *Huangdi's Inner Canon of Medicine* consists of *Fundamental Questions* and *Miraculous Pivot*; in *pinyin*, *Su Wen* and *Ling Shu*. *Su* (素) is annotated as 'plain.' *Wen* (问) means 'question.' Hence, *Su Wen* means the questions and answers of daily life. The book is a record of the daily conversations between Huangdi and his ministers such as Qibo, Shaoshi, and Bogao in the form of questions and answers. However, a physician and medical scholar named Lin Yi (林亿) in the Northern Song dynasty (960−1127) formed a different opinion after he collated medical books. He explained that according to *Qian Zao Du* (*Qián Záo Dù* 乾凿度) all things were engendered in line with the law, that is, tangibility out of intangibility; and there was a process for the development of all things: 'From supreme primordium (*tài yì* 太易), supreme origin (*tài chū* 太初), supreme beginning (*tài shǐ* 太始), to supreme simplicity (*tài sù* 太素).' Supreme primordium is the absence of *qi*; supreme origin is the origin of *qi*; supreme beginning is the beginning form of *qi*; *qi* gathers to engender the form and is called supreme simplicity. So supreme simplicity is the origin of fundamentals. Therefore, some believe *su* (素) means 'roots or fundamentals.' In this sense, *Su Wen* is translated as *Fundamental Questions*, which explores the following issues: what is the rationale behind human birth, growth, maturity, senility, and death? What are the basic principles? What is the root of life? What are the causes of diseases? And how should diseases be treated?

Ling Shu, the other part of the book, is usually translated as *Miraculous Pivot*. *Ling* (灵) means 'being efficacious.' *Shu* (枢) means 'pivot' or 'key position.' Tamba Mototane, a Japanese scholar, wrote in his *Textual Research on Chinese Medical Classics* (*Zhōng Guó Yī Jí Kǎo* 中国医籍考) that the title *Miraculous Pivot* may be related to Daoism. It makes sense because Wang Bing, who annotated *Huangdi's Inner Canon of Medicine* and gave the name *Miraculous Pivot* to the book, was a physician as well as a Daoist. If one looks at *Collected Daoist Scriptures* (*Dào Zàng* 道藏), one will come upon many similar titles containing the word 'pivot' such as *Jade Pivot* (*Yù Shū* 玉枢) and *Spirit Pivot* (*Shén Shū* 神枢).

Q5. How was the book handed down?

In the Tang dynasty, Wang Bing, whose literary name was Qixuanzi (启玄子), annotated *Fundamental Questions* with reference to the version possessed by his teacher Zhang Gong (张公). According to Wang Bing, *Huangdi's Inner Canon of Medicine* was illogically scattered and mixed up in the arrangement of contents when he came across it—the titles did not match the texts. He then spent 12 years on the rearrangement, collation, and annotation of the texts. His book *Huangdi's Inner Canon of Medicine: Fundamental Questions* was then collated by Lin Yi of the Northern Song dynasty and entitled *Huangdi's Inner Classic Fundamental Questions: Broadly Corrected and Re-annotated* (*Chóng Guǎng Bǔ Zhù Huáng Dì Nèi Jīng Sù Wèn* 重广补注黄帝内经素问). This is the widely accepted version of *Fundamental Questions* today. Wang Bing was rigorous in learning. He wrote all added words in red ink to make sure that the new and the old characters were clearly separated and would not be confused. Regrettably, when Lin Yi collated it, the commentaries were no longer shown in different colors. The old and the new characters were mixed.

Wang Bing made great contributions to the transmission of *Huangdi's Inner Canon of Medicine*. When he collated and emended *Fundamental Questions*, he referred to *Nine Volumes* (*Jiǔ Juàn* 九卷) and *Classic of Acupuncture* (*Zhēn Jīng* 针经). He combined these two books and named it *Miraculous Pivot*. Some people may ask whether *Nine Volumes*, *Classic of Acupuncture* and *Miraculous Pivot* are the same book. Based on the quotations cited in ancient literature, it is safe to say that the three books are the same.

In fact, *Miraculous Pivot* was formerly known as *Nine Volumes*. In the Eastern Han dynasty, a distinguished physician Zhang Zhongjing (张仲景) compiled a book entitled *Treatise on Cold-damage and Miscellaneous Diseases* (*Shāng Hán Zá Bìng Lùn* 伤寒杂病论). He drew upon ideas from *Fundamental Questions*, *Nine Volumes*, and *Huangdi's Eighty-one Difficult Issues*. Among them, *Nine Volumes* is referred to as *Miraculous Pivot* of the present. It was then named so because it contained nine volumes as parts of *Huangdi's Inner Canon of Medicine*. Both *Fundamental Questions* and *Miraculous Pivot* contained nine volumes respectively, making up a total of 18 volumes in *Huangdi's Inner Canon of Medicine*.

In the Jin dynasty (265–420), *Miraculous Pivot or Nine Volumes* was renamed as *Classic of Acupuncture* in *The Systematic Classic of Acupuncture and Moxibustion* (*Zhēn Jiǔ Jiǎ Yǐ Jīng* 针灸甲乙经) written by Huangfu Mi (皇甫谧), a distinguished medical scholar. Because the opening chapter of *Nine Volumes* is titled 'Nine Needles and Twelve Origins' (*Jiǔ Zhēn Shí Èr Yuán* 九针十二原) and it reads 'the acupuncture classic should be compiled first,' Huangfu Mi assumed that the book was called *Classic of Acupuncture*. In the Tang dynasty, Wang Bing changed the title of the book to *Miraculous Pivot* when he annotated *Fundamental Questions*. *Miraculous Pivot* did not receive any annotation even though it was in the revision list of the Medical Books Collation in the Northern Song dynasty. Regrettably, it later got lost in the war.

Little change had been made to Shi Song's version by later generations. It became the prototype of the printed book in the Yuan (1206–1368), Ming, and Qing (1616–1911) dynasties. In the Ming dynasty, a vassal king built a temple called Ju Jing Tang (居敬堂), in which he carved and printed *Huangdi's Inner Canon of Medicine*. It was named *Huangdi's Inner Canon of Medicine of Zhao Fu Ju Jing Tang Edition*, a very well-known edition in history.

The Ju Jing Tang edition includes both *Fundamental Questions* and *Miraculous Pivot*. This edition is the base edition of the Plum Blossom Edition today, issued by the People's Medical Publishing House in 1963. It is the best edition among all the publications of *Fundamental Questions* and *Miraculous Pivot* across the history.

Q6. What thoughts are mainly contained in the book?

Generally, four thoughts can be summarized: the holistic view, the functional perspective, the movement perspective, and the harmony or balance principle.

A. Man and nature are an integrated whole.

What one eats and wears should harmonize with the climate and seasons. This is called nurturing life in accordance with seasonal changes. TCM practitioners would prescribe different medicines for the same type of diseases. For example, it is very likely that a physician from the southern China will be different from the northern China in prescribing herbs. This is because the conditions and surroundings where patients grow up or stay are taken into account when a therapy is given. In other words, human beings and the natural world are inseparable. According to 'Fundamental Questions: Treasuring Life and Preserving Physical Appearance' (*Sù Wèn Bǎo Mìng Quán Xíng Lùn* 素问·宝命全形论), 'Man comes to life through the *qi* of heaven and earth; he matures in accordance with the laws of the four seasons.'

At the same time, man is believed to be a microcosm himself. Those who have visited Western medicine doctors may be familiar with the practice of complementing what a patient is deficient of: if deficient in sodium, iron, or potassium, one is advised to supplement the particular mineral that one needs. For instance, in the case of blood deficiency, such as severe blood loss, a blood bag containing either whole blood or platelets is required to make up for the lost blood. Nevertheless, this is not the case with TCM practice. TCM believes what one is in need of is not to be supplemented by what is outside one's body; instead, it should be engendered within one's own body. A patient with blood deficiency would be given Angelica Decoction for Tonifying Blood (*Dāng Guī Bǔ Xuè Tāng* 当归补血汤) to tonify *qi* and to generate blood. The decoction contains two herbs: Chinese Angelica (*dāng guī* 当归) and Milkvetch Root (*huáng qí* 黄芪 , or *astragalus*). Angelica mainly acts to tonify blood while astragalus mainly supplements *qi*. The decoction denotes a belief that *qi* generates blood. Angelica and astragalus are to be taken orally, acting on the human organs that can help generate blood. In this sense, the lost blood is to be made up for by the human body itself. The underlying message is—the human body is an organic whole. In TCM, five human *zang*-organs are compared to a small court, within which there are the monarch (heart), the prime minister (lung), the general (liver), the granary officer (spleen and stomach) and the labor officer (kidney). When viewed as a whole, the human body is believed to handle its internal affairs on its own when something goes wrong.

B. The human body is more of an organic whole in terms of functional performances.

Western medicine looks at the human body in an anatomical manner: it examines the specific organ itself and explores its cells. This is, however, not the case with TCM which embraces the theory of visceral manifestations (*Zàng Xiàng Theory* 藏象学说). According to Zhang Jiebin (张介宾), a commentator in the Ming dynasty, *zang* (藏) is the viscera or *zang-fu* organs hidden in the body, and *xiang* (象), the manifested changes and signs, including the observed appearance of the visceral entities. The conditions of one's viscera inside one's body are known through the signs and symptoms that are manifested outside. It is sometimes named the 'black box theory' because viscera could not be observed by the naked eye. Consequently, the concept of viscera in the TCM context is not the same as the one described in Western medicine. It makes much sense that viscera are more of an aggregate of functions in the field of TCM.

In TCM, the heart, the liver, the spleen, the lung, and the kidney are known as the five *zang*-organs while the gallbladder, the stomach, the small intestine, the large intestine, the triple energizer (*sān jiāo* 三焦) and the urinary bladder are six *fu*-organs. These five *zang*-organs and six *fu*-organs are similar to their anatomical structure from the perspective of Western medicine, among which the triple energizer is an exception: it has no counterpart in Western medicine. TCM believes that the triple energizer is similar to 'an official in charge of dredging and responsible for regulating the water passage' (Fundamental Questions: Secret Canon Stored in the Royal Library, *Sù Wèn Líng Lán Mì Diǎn Lùn* 素问·灵兰秘典论). In other words, the triple energizer is a path for the metabolism of body fluids. As far as its form is concerned, the triple energizer remains a mystery. It is quoted 'onymous but formless' in *Classic of Difficult Issues* (*Nàn Jīng* 难经).

People might wonder why TCM has achieved much success despite its obscure explanation for thousands of years in the form of *zang-fu* organs. The implication lies in the fact that TCM has a higher regard for the functions rather than the entities. *I Ching* or *Book of Changes* (*Yì Jīng* 易经) states: '*Dao* (metaphysics) is what is antecedent to the material form; *qi* (entity) is what is after the material form.' It explains that the ancient Chinese put the obscure rules and relationships in metaphysics above the specific and under-metaphysical things. They believed that things in the universe were infinite, and it was impossible to include all detailed aspects. The possible mission was to pay attention to the commonalities, that is, the extracted laws and principles.

C. The human body and the world are in constant movement.

According to *Huangdi's Inner Canon of Medicine*, physicians should always examine human life activities from the perspective of development and change. If one visits a TCM practitioner, one will be given a prescription for the ailment one has and then be told to revisit the doctor after taking three doses in three days. It is believed that the disease as well as the human body is in a state of constant change. As *Miraculous Pivot* reads: 'All diseases tend to be alleviated in the morning, are stable in the daytime, deteriorate at dusk and become severe at night.' Suppose one is having a cold, one might feel okay in the morning but sicker in the evening. For the first consultation the practitioner prescribes a patient certain herbs. A few days later, their condition may change, and it is necessary for doctors to modify prescriptions according to the changes. This practice is called syndrome or pattern differentiation and treatment: the doctor prescribes medicinals in accordance with the external manifestations of a certain disease. It is no surprise that two people with the same disease might be given different medicines or same medicines might be prescribed to patients with different diseases.

D. Harmony and balance are important principles.

Laozi (老子), a well-known ancient Chinese philosopher, once said: 'Dao begets one; out of one, two; out of two, three; and out of three, up to everything.' All things stand, facing *yang* and against *yin*. The interaction between *yin* and *yang* creates a state of harmony, and harmony in fact generates everything. According to *Huangdi's Inner Canon of Medicine*, the normal state of the human body can be described as '*yin* is stable and *yang* is compact.' In other words, *yin* and *yang* are in harmony and balance. Otherwise, diseases might occur. In TCM pathology, diseases are caused by imbalance or disharmony between *yin* and *yang*. Therefore, the regulation and treatment should be based on careful examination of *yin* and *yang*. The goal is to reach a balance.

In the opening chapter of the *Canon*, it is clearly stated that the principle of health preservation is 'abiding by the principle of *yin* and *yang*, regulating and nourishing essential *qi* with various methods and techniques of health preservation (*shù shù* 术数).' It stresses that people should follow the laws. One is the law of nature, that is, to practice health preservation according to time and place. Only by doing so can one retain harmony with nature. Another law is related to the process of human life. According to the *Canon*, the process of human life from cradle to grave can be divided into five stages—birth, growth, maturity, senility, and death, with each stage spanning ten years. When one is 10 years old, the development of the five *zang*-organs is complete; *qi* and blood flow thoroughly through the body. Children tend to run around. When one reaches the age of 20 or 30, *qi* and blood are vigorous, and the five *zang*-organs are well developed. One tends to walk quickly. In one's 30s, one tends to walk slowly. In one's 40s, the five *zang*-organs are fully developed and stability is maintained. Both body and spirit are mature. That is why Confucius states that at the age of 40, one has no doubts or misgivings. At this age, one likes to sit down. When one is 50 years old, liver *qi* begins to decline and vision begins to blur. When one is 60 years old, heart *qi* starts to decline; one is perplexed by anxiety, grief, and sorrow, which makes one sentimental. When one is in their 70s or 80s, the corporeal soul (*pò* 魄) leaves the body; one often makes mistakes while speaking and sometimes one cannot make oneself understood or tends to repeat the same thing. Since each stage of the human life has its characteristics, health preservation and treatment must be in accordance with those particular features in different life stages to attain harmony and balance.

Q7. What is the mode of thinking as is reflected in the book?

Image thinking (*xiàng sī wéi* 象思维) is the typical mode of thinking of the ancient Chinese, which is quite similar to conceptual metaphor in a sense. A case in point is as follows. When the wind blows through a tree, its leaves and branches will sway. This is called 'swaying with the wind.' The tree itself cannot take control of the swaying. As a Chinese saying goes, 'The wind will not subside even when the tree desires to stand still.' Analogically, it could be a kind of 'wind' disease if one is unable to bring his body parts under control. If you look at the patients with cerebrovascular conditions, for some of them, their hands are inflexible or even can't move. People with Parkinson's disease are found to have abnormal trembling of hands. According to TCM, it is the internal 'wind' that makes their hands tremble or stiffen, which is called predominant wind causing motion (*fēng shèng zé dòng* 风胜则动). This is an example of 'image thinking.'

Here is another example. If a kettle is to pour out the water through the spout, a small hole should be made in its lid. Only when this small hole in the lid is unobstructed can the water come out through the spout. If the hole is blocked, the water won't come out. It is precisely because of such a natural phenomenon that TCM believes the human body functions like a big kettle and the lung is like its small hole. In terms of treating edema, there is a method of ventilating the lung to relieve the inhibited urination and edema. It is specially named the lifting-off-the-lid-of-a-kettle method, an application of the mode of image thinking.

Q8. Why is it important to read the book?

Huangdi's Inner Canon of Medicine describes a set of thoughts to closely connect the human body with the natural world via the theories of *yin* and *yang*, five elements as well as essence and *qi*. It tells people a unique way of understanding, analyzing, and solving problems.

Undoubtedly, TCM has been frequently judged against the Western medical standards ever since Western medicine was introduced into China in the Ming and Qing dynasties. It seems true that what conforms to the standard of Western medicine is scientific, otherwise it is not. I'm afraid it is problematic to understand and measure the human body against a single standard because both the world and the human body are complex, and they will not be and cannot be judged by one single set of criteria. In this case, it is important to carry on TCM and stick to the way of thinking embedded in Chinese traditional culture to understand the infinite universe.

Presently, Western medicine also recognizes that individual treatment is the trend of future medical development. Psychological factors, prevention and environmental factors are to be emphasized, into which TCM does have its unique insight. In this sense, TCM can be said to represent the trend of future medical development.

Many people nowadays are talking about precision medicine and precision treatment. What is precise treatment? It can be interpreted as seeking truth from facts and treating an individual in accordance with individual condition. Isn't it a method of pattern differentiation and treatment of TCM?

Huangdi's Inner Canon of Medicine is the treasure of Chinese traditional culture and the first classic of TCM. As it is the earliest and the most comprehensive and systematic book to document the theoretical system of TCM, it lays the foundation for TCM. It is therefore called the ancestral classic and the root of medicine. Moreover, *Huangdi's Inner Canon of Medicine* reflects the way of thinking of ancient Chinese people and embodies Chinese traditional culture. It is a must-read book for those who are interested in TCM and ancient Chinese culture.

Chapter 2
The Monarch-like Heart

Q1. What does Western medicine think of the heart?

From the perspective of Western medicine, the heart is viewed as an internal organ which is situated in your left chest and pumps blood throughout your body. Inside your heart, there are valves which keep blood flowing in the right direction. When blood flows out of the heart, it carries nutrients and oxygen to all parts of your body, nourishing the organs and tissues to keep them working properly. When it flows back to the heart, blood carries waste materials such as carbon dioxide to your lungs so you can breathe it out. In this way, you have your blood cleansed.

Q2. What does TCM think of the heart?

TCM believes that the heart is not only an organ that controls blood but governs the spiritual and mental activities of the human body. According to 'Fundamental Questions: Secret Canon Stored in the Royal Library,' 'the heart is the monarch; mental and spiritual activities originate from there.' According to 'Miraculous Pivot: Pathogenic Invasion' (*Líng Shū Xié Kè* 灵枢•邪客), 'the heart is the dominator of the five *zang*-organs and the six *fu*-organs, and the residence of essence and spirit. When the heart is disturbed, the five *zang*-organs and the six *fu*-organs will be upset'. It is said in the 'Diseases' of *Classified Classics* (*Lèi Jīng* 类经) that 'the heart, being the monarch of the five *zang*-organs and the six *fu*-organs, commands the ethereal soul and the corporeal soul, and involves will.' Therefore, the heart performs the function of governing all human life activities, hence the role of the heart among the *zang-fu* organs is likened to that of the monarch of an empire.

Q3. What does the Chinese character tell us about the heart?

Figure 2-1 shows two ways of writing the word 'heart' in Chinese bronze inscriptions found on bronze wares such as tripods and plates made in the Western Zhou dynasty (1046–771 BC). On the left part of the picture, the character is purely a pictograph containing an atrium and two ventricles. On the right side, there is a dot to indicate the eyelet or opening of the heart. There is a colloquial Chinese expression *xin yanr* (*xīn yǎn ér* 心眼儿), literally heart-eye. It is commonly used to refer to mind or intelligence. For example, having *xin yanr* means having brains; having a little *xin yanr* means being narrow-minded; lack of *xin yanr* means being slow-witted; and having dead *xin yanr* means inflexibility. While the left character refers to the physical heart, the right one with a dot in it represents mind as is usually referred to for the TCM heart.

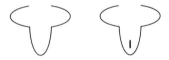

Figure 2-1   Chinese bronze inscriptions of the heart

In the Ming dynasty, a distinguished medical scholar named Li Chan (李 桤) wrote *Introduction to Medicine* (*Yī Xué Rù Mén* 医学入门), claiming there are seven openings in a heart. 'People of superior intelligence have seven openings; of mediocre intelligence, five openings; of lower intelligence, three openings; average people, two openings; fools, one little opening.' One may not survive with one little opening or orifice in the heart. Hence, the heart that the Chinese ancients discussed about involves more aspects than what the physical heart denotes. A number of Chinese characters can illustrate that the heart frequently refers to emotions and cognition, for example, fear (*kǒng* 恐), fright (*jīng* 惊), being afraid (*pà* 怕), kindness (*cí* 慈), loyalty (*zhōng* 忠), thought (*sī xiǎng* 思想), missing (*xiǎng* 想), memory (*niàn* 念), and will (*yuàn* 愿). All these characters contain the radical heart (*xīn* 心) either at the bottom or on the left side of the character.

Q4. Why is the heart compared to the monarch?

There are two reasons.

First, according to *Explanation of Scripts and Elucidation of Characters* (*Shuō Wén Jiě Zì* 说文解字 ①), 'The heart is located in the center of the human body.' No same or similar wording is found with the other *zang*-organs or *fu*-organs. It is because of this connection of the heart with the central position that comes the compound word *zhong xin* (中心, literally center-heart). Then it renders the heart to mean the core or the most essential part. The ancient Chinese attached such great importance to the heart that they regarded it as the monarch running an empire of the *zang-fu* organs. In other words, the monarch is in the center and the ministers (the other *zang-fu* organs) are peripheral.

Second, TCM believes that the heart governs consciousness, thinking, emotions and behaviors. As is mentioned in 'Fundamental Questions: Secret Canon Stored in the Royal Library', mental and spiritual activities originate from the heart. 'Miraculous Pivot: Pathogenic Invasion' states that the heart is the residence of essence and spirit. Besides, 'Fundamental Questions: Six-Plus-Six System and the Manifestations of the Viscera' (*Sù Wèn Liù Jié Zàng Xiàng Lùn* 素问·六节藏象论) states: 'The heart is the basis of life and governs the changes of spiritual and mental activities.' All these sayings support the statement that the heart governs the mind and regulates various mental activities.

---

① *Shuo Wen Jie Zi* 说文解字: the earliest dictionary of Chinese characters and one of the ancient ones in the world.

Q5. What does *shen* (神) mean?

As a key concept in TCM, *shen* (神) was believed to be the master of everything in the universe in ancient times. It is usually translated as 'spirit.' There is a well-known saying in 'Fundamental Questions: Change of Essence and Transformation of *Qi*' (*Sù Wèn Yí Jīng Biàn Qì Lùn* 素问•移精变气论): 'Those who have the spirit shall prosper; those who lose the spirit shall perish.' What is *shen* or spirit? It first refers to the phenomena of vital function in the human body. If one has the spirit, one will have bright and shining eyes, a ruddy face, natural facial expressions, clear speech, and normal behaviors. One has strength and vitality, eats, and sleeps regularly and has normal urination and bowel movements. If one loses the spirit, the following symptoms may occur: low spirits, loss of strength, dull eyes, sallow complexion, insomnia or dreaminess. In addition, *shen* refers to the higher nervous activities including consciousness, thinking, emotions, and even behaviors. As *shen*, the spiritual and mental activities of the human body, is governed by the heart, it is often referred to as the heart *shen* or heart spirit. According to 'Fundamental Questions: Secret Canon Stored in the Royal Library,' 'If the monarch does not work properly, the twelve officials will be jeopardized.' It means that the heart not only coordinates the physiological functions of all organs and tissues in the human body but also governs cognition, emotions, and volitional activities. Therefore, the heart is regarded as the monarch.

Q6. Are there any clinical cases to illustrate that the heart is the monarch?

Yes, people with epilepsy is an example. Western medicine considers epilepsy to be a neurological disorder involving temporary loss of consciousness because of abnormal electric discharge of the brain. It is characterized by the twitching of the limbs, the upward rolling of the eyes, and the strange vocal sounds. In China, it is called 'sheep-horn wind' due to the sheepish sound uttered by the patient. Sometimes, people with epilepsy may have drooling with white foam. Some may have incontinence of urination and defecation, which is the manifestation of grand mal epilepsy. Some people with epilepsy may be in a daze, drop their bowls or chopsticks while eating, which means they temporarily lose consciousness.

TCM thinks that epilepsy is caused by phlegm misting the heart orifices (*tán mí xīn qiào* 痰迷心窍), attributing its etiology and pathogenesis to the heart. Nevertheless, its signs and symptoms involve various *zang-fu* organs. Limb twitching is a sign of muscle convulsion. In TCM, convulsion is attributed to the disorder of the liver. The liver governs the eyes; therefore, when the liver does not work properly, the eyes roll upwards. The lung governs sound; therefore, when the lung has a disorder, the sound that one makes is abnormal. The kidney controls urination and defecation; therefore, when the kidney is diseased, problems with urination and defecation may occur. The spleen controls the mouth; therefore, when the spleen does not function well, the patient may have drooling with white foams. To summarize, when the heart is diseased, the other organs may suffer from malfunctions and various related signs and symptoms will occur. Hence, the heart is the monarch, governing the other *zang-fu* organs.

Q7. What will happen if the heart spirit is abnormal?

When the heart spirit is abnormal, there might be changes in one's behavior. On my way to work, I often see a man in a neighboring community, wearing a military coat and a leather hat in winter, and a wind jacket and a straw hat in summer. Sometimes he is seen directing the traffic. He is not working. In fact, he has a mental problem.

I had once a male patient who reported that he could not help walking from the city of Beijing to Tanzhe Temple①, a place of interest more than 30 kilometers away from the city center. Although he had a couple of blisters on his feet and his shoes were worn out, he kept visiting there on foot instead of taking a bus. He felt exhausted and it was painful, but he said: 'Someone ordered me to walk there.' This

---

① Tanzhe Temple: 潭柘寺, the earliest Buddhist Temple in Beijing built in the Jin dynasty (AD 265–420).

is called hallucination. There is another patient who reported that he had a time bomb in his brain, requesting the doctor to cut open his brain to take it out. If refused, he would go crazy. What is the cause of his loss of mind? It is the abnormality of his heart spirit.

The heart spirit dominates not only one's behavior, but one's body parts. It can be inferred from many idioms that are related to the heart and other body parts, for instance, *xin zhi kou kuai* (心直口快) literally the heart (is) straightforward and the mouth (speaks) fast, meaning someone is frank and outspoken; *xin ling shou qiao* (心灵手巧) literally the heart (is) clever and hands (are) deft, meaning someone is ingenious; *xin ci mian shan* (心慈面善) literally the heart (is) kind and the face (is) affable, meaning someone is kind-hearted; *xin ming yan liang* (心明眼亮) literally the heart (is) enlightened and the eyes (are) bright, meaning someone is sharp-eyed and clear-minded; *shi zhi lian xin* (十指连心) literally ten fingers are linked to the heart, meaning people are closely related to each other. These expressions indicate that the heart is tightly linked with the other parts of the body.

There are also Chinese expressions indicating that the heart spirit affects the other *zang-fu* organs. For instance, if someone is frightened and trembles with fear, it is called *xin jing dan zhan* (心惊胆战) literally the heart is frightened and the gallbladder trembles. If someone is afraid of something and cannot keep clam, it is *ti xin diao dan* (提心吊胆) literally to have the heart lifted and the gallbladder hung.

To conclude, the heart dominates the *zang-fu* organs and spirit, hence the metaphorical saying in 'Fundamental Questions: Secret Canon Stored in the Royal Library,' 'the heart is the monarch; mental and spiritual activities originate from there.'

Q8. How is health defined according to *Huangdi's Inner Canon of Medicine*?

The ancient Chinese considered health closely associated with one's heart spirit. The harmony between body and spirit is the key to health. The body and mind should be well balanced. Today, it is commonly termed as mind-body health, that is, mental health and physical health are equally important.

The World Health Organization (WHO) defines health as 'complete physical, mental and social well-being and not simply the absence of disease or infirmity.' This definition goes beyond the bio-medical model and is found to be more appropriate.

In the past, it was not rare in clinical practice that a patient would say he or she felt there was something stuck in the throat. It was impossible for them to swallow it or to spit it out. A Western medicine doctor might say there was no disorder at all after asking the patient to take a series of examinations such as using a laryngoscope and a CT scan. Then the patient resorted to a TCM doctor, saying that 'I feel there is something wrong in my throat. But I was told there was nothing wrong.'

This morbidity is termed globus hysterics. It is associated with the mind. From the perspective of TCM, it is called the binding of phlegm and *qi*. The phlegm, as TCM thinks, is intangible. A TCM doctor usually prescribes medicinals for removing phlegm and regulating *qi*. This is a case in point for the relationship between body and spirit. One's physical health is fine, but one's psychological health might be abnormal. Health involves not only physical well-being but mental and emotional well-beings. It emphasizes the role of the heart as the master of the body.

Q9. How do you nourish the heart?

The heart is a vital organ. It governs the blood circulation of the entire body. If the heart stops working, for example, because of myocardial infarction, one will not survive. To preserve health, it is of great importance to nourish the heart.

I would like to recommend an acupoint good for the heart. It is called the *nei guan* acupoint (内关穴 PC 6), a point on the palmar side of the forearm, 2 *cun* (approximately the breadth of three fingers, about 6.67 cm) above the crease of the wrist, in between the tendons of the long palmar muscle and radial flexor muscle of the wrist. The *nei guan* acupoint is in the Pericardium Meridian of Hand Reverting *Yin*. Pressing and massaging this point can bring benefits to the heart. It can relieve insomnia, vexation, irritability, palpitation, shortness of breath, chest depression, stuffiness, chest pain, and back pain. Sometimes people may feel pain in the back or in the abdomen. The backache or abdominal pain may be related to the heart problem instead of the back problem or abdominal problem. (See Figure 2-2)

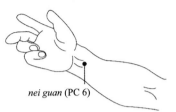

Figure 2-2 *Nei guan* acupoint

There are six main acupoints[1] for healthcare in TCM. One of them is *nei guan*, used to relieve chest and flank disorders. If one feels discomfort in the heart or in the chest, one can always massage the *nei guan* acupoint for relief. Acupuncture experiments prove that needling it can effectively improve the myocardial survival in animals with myocardial ischemia, which means massaging *nei guan* can increase blood supply to the myocardium.

How do you massage *nei guan*? You can use your thumb to massage it in a clockwise or counter-clockwise direction for about 50 times at a time. It benefits your heart and heart spirit.

---

[1] six main acupoints: including *zu san li* (足三里 ST 36), *wei zhong* (委中 BL 40), *lie que* (列缺 LU 7), *he gu* (合谷 LI 4), *nei guan* (内关 PC 6), and *shui gou* (水沟 GV 26).

Chapter 3
The Miraculous Heart Spirit

Q1. What is the pericardium?

As was previously mentioned, the heart is the monarch. If the heart is the ruler, then it should be well protected from pathogenic qi [①]. According to *Huangdi's Inner Canon of Medicine*, there are twelve *zang-fu* organs, that is, the heart, the liver, the spleen, the lung, the kidney, the gallbladder, the stomach, the large intestine, the small intestine, the triple energizer, the urinary bladder, and the pericardium. The pericardium is usually regarded as an attachment to the heart. It is also called *dan zhong* (膻中) and serves as the wall to guard the heart. Hence, 'Miraculous Pivot: Pathogenic Invasion' states that various pathogenic factors would attack the pericardium instead of the heart because the former is the protective wall of the latter. Imagine when the emperor is confronted with danger, the attendant by his side would rise to protect. That is why the pericardium is described as the royal courtier who is responsible for happiness and joy in the 'Fundamental Questions: Secret Canon Stored in the Royal Library.'

[①] pathogenic *qi*: opposite of healthy *qi*, referring to all kinds of pathogenic factors, including those in the external environment and those inside the body.

Q2. What are the four aspects related to the heart spirit?

Vital functions are governed by the heart spirit. If vital functions are normal, the heart spirit is normal. They come and go together. That is why 'Fundamental Questions: Change of Essence and Transformation of *Qi*' states: 'Those who have the spirit shall prosper; those who lose the spirit shall perish.' In addition to vital functions, the heart spirit contains the following four aspects.

First, the heart spirit affects one's thoughts and personal qualities. Here is a legendary story about Bianque (扁鹊)[①] transplanting the hearts for two people. It is said that Gong Hu (公扈) of the State of Lu and Qi Ying (齐婴) of the State of Zhao went to visit Bianque when they felt ill, and both regained health after the treatment. Bian Que said to them: 'The two of you got sick due to the invasion of external pathogens. After you took the medicine I prescribed to you, the external pathogenic factors are removed, and your health is restored. But you two have the problems that you are born with, and it is difficult to relieve them.' According to Bianque, Gong Hu was good at thinking but had a weak temperament and was indecisive. That is, Gong Hu had more resourcefulness than courage. Qi Ying was just the opposite. He was arbitrary and bold enough to fight and kill, but he was short of wit. That is, Qi Ying had more courage than wisdom. Upon hearing it, the two asked what they could do. Bianque then said: 'The heart dominates spirit. I'll have your hearts exchanged.' They agreed. So, Bianque gave them anesthetic medicine and made both of them unconscious for three days. During that time, Bianque opened their chests, exchanged their hearts, and applied a magic medicinal for their recovery after sewing up the incisions. A few days later, the two regained consciousness and health, feeling they were both brave and resourceful. Upon returning home, however, they went to the other's house instead of their own. Neither recognized his wife or children. Both men went to the state court to sue each other. They were not pacified until Bianque was invited to explain what had happened. This story was recorded in a book named *Liezi* (*Liè Zǐ* 列子). It attempts to demonstrate that the heart governs spirit

---

① Bianque (扁鹊): a mythical TCM doctor with supernatural capabilities.

which includes one's temperament or personality. It also includes one's memories or thoughts. Otherwise, how come the two men went to the other's house instead of their own house? To conclude, thoughts and temperaments are considered to be associated with the heart.

Modern stories also prove this argument. It was reported in a newspaper a couple of years ago that a woman transplanted with the heart of a young man who died of a motor accident experienced great changes in her temperament. Before the heart transplant, she was mild and gentle. After having the new heart, however, she became aggressive and violent. In addition, she liked to smoke cigarettes and drink wine. Similar stories of temperament change after the heart transplant can also be found in some movies such as *21 Grams* (2003) and *The Devil Inside Me* (2011). In the first movie, the main character Paul Rivers, starring Sean Penn, had the memory and personality of the donor after a man's heart was transplanted into his chest. Recent articles also report personality changes following heart transplantation and discuss the transfer of cellular memory from the donor to the recipient. Nevertheless, it requires further research whether these accounts provided evidence to support the TCM theory that the heart governs spirit. The legendary story of Bianque exchanging the hearts is meant to say that the transplanted heart is not the heart in the Western medical sense. It refers to the heart within the TCM scope.

Second, the heart spirit affects emotions. Such emotions as joy, anger, anxiety, overthinking, sorrow, fear, and fright are all related to the heart. Among them, joy is most closely connected with the heart. The other emotions such as anger, overthinking, sorrow, and fright are most closely connected with the liver, the spleen, the lung, and the kidney, respectively. (See Table 3-1)

Table 3-1   *Zang*-organs with their corresponding elements, colors, and emotions

Zang-organs	Elements	Colors	Emotions
heart	fire	red	joy
liver	wood	green	anger
spleen	earth	yellow	overthinking (and anxiety)
lung	metal	white	sorrow
kidney	water	black	fright (and fear)

Joy is a pleasant thing. It renders the smooth flow of *qi*. According to 'Fundamental Questions: Pain' (*Sù Wèn Jǔ Tòng Lùn* 素问·举痛论), 'Joy makes *qi* harmonious and mind unimpeded.' However, excessive joy slackens *qi*. When one becomes excessively joyous, heart *qi* scatters and one might be out of one's mind.

There is a well-known story of Fan Jin (范进) passing the imperial examination in *The History of Confucian School* [①] (*Rú Lín Wài Shǐ* 儒林外史). In the Ming dynasty there was a poor scholar named Fan Jin. He had taken the annual imperial examination ever since he was 20 years old, but he failed repeatedly. He was jeered and looked down upon by his folk people. When he was 54 years old, Fan Jin took the examination again and was told by the messenger that he succeeded this time. He could not believe his ears, and then became wild with joy. He clapped his hands, extremely thrilled, and then suddenly fell to the ground, unconscious. After his mother fed him some water, he came to life. He shouted: 'I made it... I made it...' and dashed out of his house. It was raining hard. He slipped and fell, crawled, stood up and ran in the rain, making himself wet and dirty all over the body. To people's surprise, the news made Fan Jin so excited that he went crazy. This is a case in point for the saying: excessive joy impairs the heart, leading to the scattering of heart *qi* and abnormal thinking ability.

Among the seven emotions—joy, anger, anxiety, overthinking, sorrow, fear and fright, joy is perhaps the only one that is positive and beneficial to the human body. Hence, Mr. Hou Baolin (侯宝林), a master of the cross-talk art in China, suggested that hospitals have a cross-talk department to entertain the patients. Perhaps laughter makes patients feel better and relieves their sufferings. As the Chinese saying goes, mirth makes one younger. Mirth is surely good to people. It is, therefore, of great importance to keep a positive mentality for the sake of health preservation and disease prevention. If one is happy every day, one will maintain smooth and gentle flow of *qi* and blood and one can avoid diseases or somehow have illnesses relieved.

Emotions are related to the condition of the heart. It is repeatedly highlighted in 'Miraculous Pivot: Symptoms of *Zang-fu* Organs Due to the Invasion of Pathogenic

---

[①] *The History of Confucian School*: a well-known satirical novel written by Wu Jingzi (吴敬梓) of the Qing dynasty (1616–1911), which initiates the direct evaluation of reality in the form of stories.

Qi' (*Líng Shū: Xié Qì Zàng Fǔ Bìng Xíng* 灵枢•邪气脏腑病形) that anxiety and fear also impair the heart. Various emotions, for instance, anxiety, fear, and fright will harm the human body if they are in excess. When people nurture their life, they ought to nurture their emotions.

Third, the heart spirit affects perception. According to 'Miraculous Pivot: Basic State of Spirit' (*Líng Shū Běn Shén* 灵枢•本神), 'What helps people perceive things is called the heart spirit.' That is, the heart is responsible for perceiving external stimuli and information. Perception is therefore part of the job of the heart spirit. When the perception of body goes wrong, it can be treated from the aspect of the heart.

The treatment of a patient by my mentor, Prof. Wang Hongtu (王洪图), left me a deep impression. A female patient in her early 50s visited his consultation room dozens of years ago when I was an intern there. She complained that she had a generalized itching and pain in her body. She felt so miserable that she even wanted to commit suicide. She told us that her girdle was like a straw rope tied to her naked waist. She had to wear her clothes inside out. If not, once the seams of clothes touched her body, she would feel itchy and painful. She had consulted many doctors and all prescribed therapies had resulted in failure. Prof. Wang said that her disease was a kind of dysfunction of perception related to the heart. According to the well-known 19 mechanisms of diseases discussed in 'Fundamental Questions: Significant Discussions on the Most Important and Abstruse Theory' (*Sù Wèn Zhì Zhēn Yào Dà Lùn* 素问•至真要大论), 'All pains, itches and sores are ascribed to the heart.' That is, patients with pains, itches, sores, or ulcers can be treated from the aspect of the heart. For these signs and symptoms, the therapy of clearing the heart heat, cooling blood, and activating blood circulation is the way to address the problem and it brings very good results. Medicinals can include Golden Thread (*huáng lián* 黄连), Tree Peony Bark (*dān pí* 丹皮), Red Peony Root (*chì sháo* 赤芍), Cape-Jasmine Fruit (*zhī zǐ* 栀子), and Danshen Root (*dān shēn* 丹参).

The above case is an illustration of the physical perception. One may perceive pains and itches or feel there is something stuck in the throat, difficult to swallow it or to spit it out.

There is another type of perception: mental. Here is a different case of a newly-wedded female teacher in her 30s. She complained that she did not dare to walk beside the tall buildings. She was afraid that someone might throw things from high above and she would become the victim. As a result of anxiety and fear, she had insomnia, irregular menstruation and was in low spirits. She had to stop teaching. This is another example of the heart-spirit problem.

Fourth, the heart spirit affects sleep. Sleep is part of one's everyday life, approximately taking up seven or eight hours out of twenty-four hours a day for average adults. One cannot survive if deprived of sleep for a long time. Sleep is an essential part of normal physiological activity. Through sleep, the human body gets rest, and the spirit and physical strength are fully recharged. Based on the observation of human and nature and combined with the movement of celestial bodies and the alternation of day and night, *Huangdi's Inner Canon of Medicine* describes the movement of *qi* and blood in meridians and the function of *zang-fu* organs. 'Miraculous Pivot: Great Perplexity' (*Líng Shū Dà Huò Lùn* 灵枢•大惑论) states that 'Defense *qi* is what circulates in the *yang* aspect in the daytime and in the *yin* aspect at night.' The movement of nutrient *qi* and defense *qi* is not only directly affected by the day-night alternation, but it affects people's sleep. For example, 'Miraculous Pivot: Questions and Answers' (*Líng Shū Kǒu Wèn* 灵枢•口问) states: 'Defense *qi* circulates in the *yang* aspect in the daytime and in the *yin* aspect at night. *Yin* dominates night. Night governs sleep. When *yang qi* is exhausted, *yin qi* will be predominant. Therefore, people close eyes to sleep. When *yin qi* is exhausted, *yang qi* will be predominant. Therefore, people remain awake.'

It can be seen from *Huangdi's Inner Canon of Medicine* that the movement of *yang qi* and *yin qi* is directly affected by the day-night alternation and corresponds to nature. It determines one's sleep-wake cycle. In plain language, at the daytime, *yang qi* is predominant which governs mobility; hence at the daytime people usually engage in different activities such as thinking, work, and movement. After the sun sets and it gets dark, night falls. At the nighttime, *yin qi* is dominant which governs stillness; hence at night people usually stop working or thinking and go to sleep.

Sleep is regarded as a normal physiological activity according to Western medicine. Sleep disorders are not attributed to mental or spiritual illness. In the field of TCM, however, sleep is thought to be governed by the heart spirit. Sleep disorders such as insomnia, difficulty in falling asleep or somnambulism are attributed to the dysfunction of the heart spirit.

There are a variety of sleep disorders.

The first type is sleeplessness. People with insomnia usually have a hard time falling asleep despite their efforts of counting sheep, listening to soothing music or reading a novel. They toss and turn in bed, trying to sleep.

The second type is difficulty in maintaining sleep, that is, when people wake up during the sleep it is hard for them to resume sleep.

The third type is parasomnias. For example, some people talk continuously during their sleep without being aware of it, disturbing other people in the same room. In severe cases, some people may get up and walk around while in a state of sleep. I heard of a sleepwalker saying that he got up to wash his hands during his sleep. He did not use the bathroom inside his bedroom because his wife was sleeping and he did not want to wake her up, so he sleepwalked to the living room, went to the other bathroom, turned on the light and the tap. He did not wake up until the cool water flowed into his palms. He then realized that he was dreaming of washing hands during his sleep. According to TCM doctors, disturbed heart spirit contributes to sleepwalking. The heart fails to house its spirit. To be more specific, the ethereal soul that is chiefly housed by the liver left its residence. The ethereal soul corresponds to the higher aspect of perception. When the perception is not governed by the heart spirit and leaves its residence, disorders then occur.

The fourth type is excessive sleepiness. Some people have difficulty staying awake during the daytime. A patient reported that he was asleep while riding his bike and did not wake up even when he fell into a ditch. Another patient, a young driver, reported that he had to sleep long hours during the night. But at nine o'clock of the following morning, he would feel sleepy again. He had an accident resulting in bone fracture and had to end his driving career.

One day, when I was about to end a day's work and left for home, a 40-year-old man came to my consultation room. He bowed to me, asking me for medical help. He complained that he had had difficulty falling asleep for years despite sleeping pills. However, his family member who accompanied him clarified that he could actually sleep for a while after he took sleeping pills. Nevertheless, the patient felt that he had been awake all the time and been aware of whatever was taking place around him. He felt rather miserable and was tense and anxious. This is also a case of the heart-spirit disorder.

Q3. How do TCM doctors address sleep disorders?

Sleep disorders are considered to be associated with the heart-spirit problem. It is common for TCM doctors to prescribe medicines that can pacify the mind and calm the spirit. One is also advised to eat more food of *yin* nature and avoid food of *yang* nature to nourish *qi* and blood. But remember, sleep disorders such as insomnia is a complex issue. The best strategy is to visit the doctor and appropriate treatment should be given based on syndrome or pattern differentiation.

Q4. Are there any well-known Chinese herbal formulas for sleep disorders?

There is a well-known formula named *Jiao Tai* Pill (*Jiāo Tài Wán* 交泰丸) that is sometimes translated as Communicating and Tranquilizing Pill. It was documented in *Han's General Medicine* (*Hán Shì Yī Tōng* 韩氏医通) written by Han Mao (韩懋) of the Ming dynasty. It contains only two ingredients: Golden Thread and Cassia Bark (*ròu guì* 肉桂). Golden Thread is believed to enter the heart meridian. Bitter in taste and cold in nature, it is used to clear heat and purge fire. Its medicinal action goes downward. Cassia Bark enters the kidney meridian. Pungent in taste and hot in nature, it is used to warm the kidney. According to the five-element theory, the heart corresponds to fire and the kidney to water. Therefore, the use of Golden Thread reduces fire and makes it move downward. The use of Cassia Bark warms water and makes it go upward. In this way, water and fire meet and it is called water-fire coordination, or in terms of their corresponding organs, kidney-heart interaction.

Why is the formula named *Jiao Tai* Pill? *Tai* (泰) refers to the *Tai* hexagram. In *Book of Changes*, there is a very good hexagram, the *Tai* hexagram, and a very bad one, the *Pi* (否) hexagram. The *Pi* hexagram contains the *Qian* (乾) hexagram (heaven) in the upper part and the *Kun* (坤) hexagram (earth) in the lower part. The *Qian* hexagram is made up of straight unbroken lines, which represents *yang*. The *Kun* hexagram is made up of broken lines, which represents *yin*. *Yang* ascends while *yin* descends. Therefore, as the *Pi* hexagram shows, *yin* and *yang* will never ever interact. If *yin* and *yang* fail to interact or communicate, myriad things will not be engendered because according to *Huangdi's Inner Canon of Medicine* things in the nature are generated because of the interaction of heaven-*qi* and earth-*qi*. In Chinese, *pi* means bad and obstructed and it symbolizes ominousness. The *Tai* hexagram, however, is just the opposite. It contains the *Kun* hexagram (earth, *yin*) in the upper part and the *Qian* hexagram (heaven, *yang*) in the lower part. Hence, *yin* (going down) and *yang* (going up) will meet and interact. As a result, myriad beings will come to life. In Chinese, *tai* means peace and stability which is a good sign. Hence, *Jiao Tai* Pill is aimed to bring together water and fire and creates a harmonious state. (See Figure 3-1 and Figure 3-2)

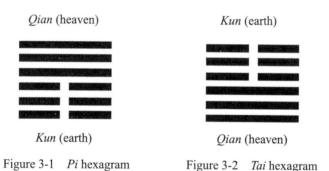

Qian (heaven)	*Kun* (earth)
Kun (earth)	*Qian* (heaven)
Figure 3-1 *Pi* hexagram	Figure 3-2 *Tai* hexagram

Jiao Tai Pill is widely used in clinical practice with modification and development. It is proposed that fire (heart) and water (kidney) interact in the middle energizer (spleen and stomach). Based on this view, sleep disorders can also be relieved via the treatment for the spleen and the stomach. In sum, different therapeutic methods can be adopted based on pattern differentiation. To relieve insomnia, medicinals for calming the spirit or reducing (heart) fire or nourishing (kidney) water or harmonizing the spleen and the stomach can be the options according to the manifested signs and symptoms. There is a saying: 'The spleen is the yellow matchmaker for the interaction of water and fire.' According to the relationship between the five elements and the five colors, the spleen corresponds to yellow, hence the yellow matchmaker. That is, the spleen and the stomach play an important part in the communication of the heart and the kidney. Just as what is said in 'Fundamental Questions: Disharmony' (*Sù Wèn Nì Tiáo Lùn* 素问·逆调论): 'Stomach-qi disharmony disturbs sleep.' In this quote, the stomach does not refer to the physical stomach only; it also involves the spleen, because both the spleen and the stomach responsible for the transportation and transformation of food and water (or metabolism) belong to the middle energizer and they are interior-exteriorly related.

TCM believes that the disharmony between the spleen and the stomach may lead to insomnia. It is due to the obstruction in the communication between the heart and the kidney. Once the obstruction is removed, that is, the spleen and the stomach are harmonious, the communication between the heart and the kidney will be smooth. Then insomnia is cured. For the treatment of insomnia, one related herbal formula was recorded out of a total of 13 in *Huangdi's Inner Canon of Medicine*: Pinellia Tuber and Broomcorn Millet Decoction (*Bàn Xià Shú Mǐ Tāng* 半夏秫米 汤). Pinellia Tuber (*bàn xià* 半夏) is bitter in flavor and warm in property. It can strengthen the spleen, dry dampness, and resolve phlegm to eliminate fullness. Broomcorn Millet (*shú mǐ* 秫米) is sweet in flavor and slightly cold in property. It can promote the function of the stomach and the intestines, clear depressed heat, reduce *yang* and tonify *yin*. The combination of the cold herb and the warm herb allows the reinforcement of the spleen and the harmonization of the stomach. It is beneficial to the removal of the obstruction and thus facilitates the communication between the heart and the kidney. In this way, insomnia is relieved. Pinellia Tuber and Broomcorn Millet Decoction is used to dredge the passage and regulate *yin* and *yang*. It is, as described in *Huangdi's Inner Canon of Medicine*, so effective that patients may fall asleep the moment they put down the cup of medicine.

There is another formula for insomnia called Golden Thread and Donkey-hide Glue Decoction (*Huáng Lián Ē Jiāo Tāng* 黄连阿胶汤). The therapy is mainly targeted at kidney deficiency, hence donkey-hide glue is used to nourish kidney *yin*. Golden Thread and Baical Skullcap Root (*huáng qín* 黄芩) are used to clear heat, drain dampness, and purge fire.

To sum up, different therapies will be used for the same disease (insomnia). One should remember not to simply turn to a well-known prescription for cure. It is of vital importance that pattern differentiation and treatment are always necessary.

Q5. Is sleeplessness a normal part of life?

It is a misunderstanding that sleeplessness is not a disease. Some people think that one cannot fall asleep because one is not sleepy enough. Perhaps only the sufferers know how miserable they are. If one is deprived of sleep for a period of time, one can experience anxiety, weight loss, and problems with concentration and memory. Overall health can be impaired. If these signs and symptoms occur, one should seek medical treatment without delay.

Sleep provides nutrition to health. Li Yu (李渔), also known as Li Liweng (李笠翁), a Chinese playwright of the Qing dynasty, states that for health preservation, sleep is of utmost priority. It makes much sense. For children, sleep is of enormous importance to their growth and brain development. Without enough sleep, certain cognitive functions might not work as effectively as they should have. For women, sleep is said to have beautifying function. No makeup is better than sufficient sleep. Sleep helps the human body repair, regenerate, and recover. That is why when one has a cold, one is always told to have a good rest or sleep so that one's resistance against the disease can be improved.

Q6. What food is good for sleep?

TCM thinks that medicine and food are of the same origin. Instead of taking Spine Date Seed Drink for Calming Spirit (*Zǎo Rén Ān Shén Yè* 枣仁安神液), one can take Chinese rice porridge of Spine Date Seed (*suān zǎo rén* 酸枣仁) to help sleep. Spine Date Seed is a good tranquilizer. Sweet and sour in taste and neutral in property, it is commonly used to relieve fidgetiness, palpitation, and insomnia. One can buy some Spine Date Seeds from the drugstore or supermarket, boil them, and remove the residues. Then one can use the remaining soup to make congee. Eating Spine Date Seed Congee can benefit the (liver) blood and nourish the (heart) spirit.

Chapter 4
The Key to Emotional Regulation

Q1. Why is cultivating spirit of utmost importance to nourishing the heart?

According to TCM, the heart is something beyond the physical heart. It not only pumps blood but governs spirit, consciousness, and thinking which are the powers of the human body. The heart spirit, or in short, spirit, controls the *zang-fu* organs and the physical activities of the body. Since spirit has tremendous effects on health, the ancient Chinese placed great emphasis on spirit cultivation when they put forth the principles for health preservation or life nurturing.

Q2. What does *Huangdi's Inner Canon of Medicine* say about cultivating spirit?

There is a well-quoted line in the opening chapter of the book: '*tian dan xu wu, zhen qi cong zhi, jing shen nei shou, bing an cong lai* (恬惔虚无, 真气从之, 精神内守, 病安从来).' *Tian* (恬) means quietness; *dan* (惔) means simplicity; *xu wu* (虚无) means nothingness, that is, being free from all wants and desires. The direct translation of the whole sentence would be: 'keep placidity and nothingness, and healthy *qi* in the body will be in harmony, spirit will remain inside. If so, how can diseases occur?' To put it in a simple way, 'uncluttered mind preserves vitality; good spirit alienates fatality.'[①]

For spirit cultivation, the top priority is to maintain inner peace, abstaining from excessive wants and desires. To quote another line in the opening chapter, 'Wills should be controlled, and desires should be reduced (*zhì xián ér shǎo yù* 志闲 而少欲).' According to *Explanation of Scripts and Elucidation of Characters*, the character 闲 (*xián*) is made up of a door (门) and wood (木), and it is explained in *Various Rhymes (Guǎng Yùn 广韵*[②]) that *xian* means prevention or control. In other words, one should exercise restraint of their wants and desires, taking a humble and compatible attitude, being indifferent to fame or wealth, and being detached and refined to avoid experiencing negative emotions. In doing so, one can maintain a tranquil mind and keep the spirit in its place so that *zang-fu* organs as well as *qi* and blood can be regulated, free flow of *qi* can be attained, *yin* and *yang* can remain stable and compact, and body-spirit harmony can be achieved. Thus, one enjoys health and longevity.

Q3. What are the three ways of cultivating spirit?

Cultivating spirit involves the following three aspects: regulating mindset, regulating emotions, and venting emotions. Questions 4–6 provide more details.

Q4. How do you regulate mindset?

Let me begin with a story. Huangdi asked his teacher Guangchengzi (广成子)[③]

---

① Cited from Xie, Zhufan & Xie, Fang. *Classified Dictionary of Traditional Chinese Medicine* [M]. 2nd new edition. Beijing: Foreign Languages Press, 2019: 507.

② *Guǎng Yùn* 广韵 : a representative work on phonetics in the middle ancient times, having a lot of Chinese characters with other pronunciations.

③ Guangchengzi (广成子): a legendary figure in Daoism and the teacher of Huangdi.

about how to nurture life. As you may know, Guangchengzi was a master who was well versed in how to preserve health. He was an immortal and often rode on the back of his crane wandering around, imparting his knowledge of how to live a long life. Guangchengzi said to Huangdi: 'If you can refrain from seeing or listening to what exists external to yourself or from having something on your mind, you can achieve the goal of health preservation and longevity.' In other words, you should see, hear, or think of no things. Then you may keep a tranquil mind and have a good mindset.

There are generally three ways to regulate mindset.

First, do not aim too high. You should set your goal in a realistic manner. It does not necessarily mean that you should not have a long-term goal. The hidden message is that you could divide your long-term goal into several smaller tasks, possible for gradual achievement. In this way, you will feel happy about what you have achieved.

For example, some time ago, I was invited to lecture for a two-week training program at Tsinghua University. Some trainees came to Beijing from remote areas such as Yunnan, Guizhou, and the other places of China. When the program was about to end, some of them were very happy because they were to return home and meet their beloved ones before long. Some otherwise felt a little anxious. If you asked them why they were anxious, they said they would have a lot of work to do and a lot of things to deal with after they finished the course and returned home. Different mindset gives different response. If one could set this two-week program as the goal, once it is over and one goes home, then one would be very happy and content. Therefore, big goals have to be broken down into smaller ones. Lofty ideals are necessary. But one can make such schedules as what one has to do this week, the following week, the week after the next and so on. One can finish work week by week and approach the goal bit by bit. Just as what the ancient Chinese say: 'if one does not accumulate steps, one cannot reach a thousand miles. If streams are not accumulated, rivers or seas will never ever come into being.'

Second, do not get caught up in comparison. When one compares with others, one is likely to compare their weaknesses with the strengths of others. In this way, one is deemed to feel depressed. No one is perfect. But everyone has their own specific sets of strengths. If one can make good use of their capabilities and play to their strengths, success will not be far away from them.

People undertake different jobs and shoulder different responsibilities. For instance, chances are that business people earn more money. They may dress in expensive clothes, live in villas, or drive luxury cars. But they have to work longer hours. Quite a lot of Chinese business people including presidents, general managers, and managers of companies or corporations attend Master of Business Administration (MBA) or Executive Master of Business Administration (EMBA) training programs because they feel they need to acquire new knowledge and obtain a degree. Another example is that when there is a dangerous event, there will be journalists or reporters. It is hard and tiring for them to show up and provide timely reports. On the other hand, while average people have few opportunities to travel at home or abroad, journalists have more chances to see the outside world. To cite one more example, some people are not only administrators but also professionals. The principal and the dean of the school, for example, not only do administrative work but shoulder teaching responsibilities. They have to work extremely hard, and they do not have as much time and energy for improving their expertise as the ordinary teaching staff otherwise do. This is their weakness. However, as administrators, they are involved in decision making and it is likely that they have many people following them. This is what ordinary teachers cannot enjoy. It is evident that people have both strengths and weaknesses of their own. If you really want to compare with others, it is suggested that you compare your strengths with the weaknesses of others.

Several years before, I read a short story on WeChat[①]. A child received 80 points out of 100 points in his math test. When his father took his paper and looked at it, he was very upset. He said to his son: 'Look at Xiao Gang next door. He got full marks in the math test. How did you only get 80 points? How could you be so stupid? Why can't you put enough effort into learning?' Upon hearing it, his son, after pondering for a moment, said to his father: 'Daddy, there is a villa not far from our house. Its owner is the president of a company. Why are you just a tiny director of a department? Why do we have to live in this two-bedroom apartment?' His father was astounded. As you may realize, it is important for people to adjust mindset.

---

① WeChat: a popular messaging and social media App in China.

In the opening chapter of the *Canon*, 'Fundamental Questions: Genuine *Qi* Endowed by Heaven in Remote Antiquity' (*Sù Wèn Shàng Gǔ Tiān Zhēn Lùn* 素问·上古天真论), it is emphasized that people in remote antiquity did not care whether one held a high position or a low position but lived simply and naturally. Refrain yourself from comparing to others. If you want to, you'd better compare what you are with what you were, compare what you have achieved with what you had once failed in.

Third, take the initiative to find fun in life. Some people think it is not easy to have fun. It is surely fun if you can paint a Chinese painting, play Go and/or practice calligraphy. Doing those things takes up time and effort. But there are some easy things to do for fun. For example, it can be joyous to sit down watching two or three episodes of your favorite TV series, or to invite a couple of your friends for a cup of coffee or an outing from time to time. Whether it sounds vulgar or decent, it can be called the fun in life as long as you enjoy it. When you have your desires satisfied, you will be content with who you are and what you have.

Q5. How do you regulate emotions?

There are seven emotions in TCM, namely joy, anger, anxiety, overthinking, sorrow, fear, and fright. Among them, joy is seemingly the only positive emotion that benefits the human body. It is joy that can help with the smooth flow of *qi* and blood, permitting the normal function of the heart spirit so that the heart spirit can properly govern one's physical and mental activities. In this sense, one needs to find more fun and joy in daily life.

There is a story in 'Zhuangzi: Enjoyment in Untroubled Ease' (*Zhuāng Zǐ Xiāo Yáo Yóu* 庄子·逍遥游) about a sparrow and a mythological giant bird called Peng (鹏) or roc. One day when the sparrow is flying, it finds a cloud floating above it. It is the Peng towering above it. Legends say that the back of the Peng is like Mount Tai[①] and its wings are like clouds upon the border of the sky. Its flight is only made

---

①   Mount Tai: one of the five Great Mountains in China, located north of Tai'an city in Shandong province.

possible when it ascends extremely high above the sky. Mao Zedong (毛泽东)[①] describes the Peng in one of his poems entitled 'Two Birds: A Dialogue—to the tune of Nian Nu Jiao'[②]. It reads as follows:

> The roc wings fanwise,
>
> Soaring ninety thousand *li*
>
> And rousing a raging cyclone.
>
> The blue sky on his back, he looks down
>
> To survey Man's world with its towns and cities.

Looking at the Peng, the sparrow thinks to itself: 'You are so huge and you fly so high above. Isn't it simply flying as I do in the sky? Although I fly low, I am free. I fly from this locust to that elm. If I'm tired of flying, I can take a rest in the bush and then fly about. Can you have a break in the middle of your flight? I'm afraid it is not easy. During my flight, if I do not feel well or feel sick, I might fall and only make a small pit in the ground. What if you fall on the ground? Well, I am no different from you in terms of freedom and ease.' Nonetheless, it is not uncommon for people to sing for the Peng and condemn the sparrow. This shows different mentality.

The story about the two birds reminds me of an anecdote. There is an official in charge of education administration in a certain part of the country. He once paid a visit to a middle school in a remote area for an investigation. There he came across a teacher who was fresh out of college. When he visited the room of the young teacher, he caught sight of a calligraphy scroll which read 'sparrow in the bush.' The official asked the young teacher: 'Don't you want to aim high and make progress after graduating from university? If your students come to your room and see the calligraphy, won't the negative emotion infect them?' The implicature is definite: the young man lacks ambition; he should take off the scroll. Soon after, the teacher was transferred to a different administration area. Later, the official was told that the teacher was somewhat dissatisfied with him. The official then consulted the

---

① Mao Zedong (毛泽东): the first Chinese leader who announced the founding of the People's Republic of China at Tian'anmen Square in October, 1949.

② Cited from Mao Zedong (1976) *Two Birds: A Dialogue* (Autumn 1965), Chinese Law & Government, 9:1–2, 107–108, DOI: 10.2753/CLG0009-4609090102107.

book *Zhuangzi* (*Zhuāng Zǐ* 庄子) and read the dialogue between the Peng and the sparrow. 'Perhaps in such a remote place', the official reflected, 'it would have been very difficult for the young man to cope with things even if he had had a lofty mind.' Perhaps there were few things he could do when he could not foresee the silver lining of a cloud as was described by Lu You (陆游) of the Southern Song dynasty: 'Over numerous mountains and streams I had my doubts that I could find the road. Then out of the shade of the willows came bright flowers and another village.'[①] In this case, it might not have been a bad strategy for the young man to adopt the carefree lifestyle of the little sparrow. Otherwise, he might have suffered from depression. From this perspective, what the young teacher did was reasonable.

The thought of regulating the mindset discussed above is derived from Zhuangzi (庄子), a pivotal figure in Daoism along with Laozi (老子). The two of them are usually called Lao-Zhuang. Some of the thoughts in *Huangdi's Inner Canon of Medicine* can be traced to the Lao-Zhuang thought, that is, the thought of non-action. Non-action does not mean doing nothing. It means people should not intentionally seek anything but follow the rules of nature. There are a variety of natural laws, for instance, the seasonal changes and the process of human life from cradle to grave (in TCM from birth to growth, maturity, senility, and finally death). Therefore, following the laws of nature is the first necessity of nurturing life, as is stated in 'Fundamental Questions: Genuine *Qi* Endowed by Heaven in Remote Antiquity,' 'one should abide by the natural law of *yin* and *yang*.'

The second method of emotional regulation can be called 'one emotion conquering another.' It is a way to restrain one emotion by stimulating another to break the vicious circle and thus treat emotional disorders. In the Yuan dynasty (1206–1368), there was a well-known physician named Zhu Danxi (朱丹溪)[②]. He was adept at using one emotion to relieve another which was in excess and causing disorder. One day he was asked to treat a female patient who had no desire for eating or talking and who was somewhat depressed. She lay in her bed facing the wall all

---

①   Cited from Touring Shanxi Village – Wikisource, the free online library, available at https://en.wikisource.org/wiki/Translation:Touring_Shanxi_Village.

②   Zhu Danxi (朱丹溪): the author of *Danxi's Experiential Therapy* (*Dān Xī Xīn Fǎ* 丹溪心法) whose main doctrine is that *yang* is often excessive, and *yin* is often deficient.

day long and refused to communicate with anyone. Her father had consulted many physicians for a cure, but no effective results had been obtained before he finally turned to Zhu Danxi for help. Zhu examined the patient, asked a few questions, took her pulse, and then said that her pulse at *cun kou* (寸口)[1] was wiry. According to TCM theory, wiry pulse indicates liver-*qi* stagnation, that is, liver *qi* is obstructed and fails to flow smoothly. Zhu Danxi suspected that her illness was due to excessive thinking. When asked, her father said that soon after her marriage her husband had been away to work and had not returned home ever since. Moreover, for two years, she had not received any single message or letter from her husband. It was evident that the young woman fell ill because of her excessive thinking of her husband. Long-term yearning caused lovesickness. That was why she was depressed and did not feel like eating, drinking, or talking.

How did Zhu Danxi treat her? He offered her father an idea. After her father understood it, he drove his daughter into a rage. On the following day, his daughter began to eat congee and have meals. Though still annoyed, she began to talk with others. Her father went to see Zhu Danxi again. The latter said that she was improving but another round of treatment was yet necessary. According to Zhu, her *qi* was no longer knotted and started to flow smoothly. But it was still possible for her *qi* to rebind. To prevent the re-stagnation of *qi*, they claimed that her husband had written her a letter in which he told her that he would be coming home in two months. The woman was very happy at the news. To her joy, her husband did come back soon, and her illness was then cured. This is a case in point for the therapy of one emotion conquering another.

According to TCM, emotions are governed by the heart and each of the emotions is closely connected to a specific *zang*-organ (and its corresponding element). Specifically, joy is related to the heart (fire), anger to the liver (wood), overthinking to the spleen (earth), sorrow and anxiety to the lung (metal), and fear and fright to the kidney (water). Among the five elements, there exists a relationship of restriction, which means one element restricts and brings another element under control. It follows the sequence below: wood restricts earth; earth restricts

---

①   *cun kou* (寸口): the usual region on the wrist for taking the pulse of radial artery.

water; water restricts fire; fire restricts metal; and metal restricts wood. In terms of emotions, the sequence is: anger conquers thought; thought conquers fear; fear conquers joy; joy conquers sorrow; and sorrow conquers anger. In other words, the disorder caused by excessive thought can be treated with the method of making the patient angry; the illness caused by excessive fear can be relieved via making the patient indulge in thinking, and so on. To sum up, the method of one emotion conquering another is used in accordance with the following principles: joy impairs the heart, but fear conquers joy; overthinking impairs the spleen, but anger conquers overthinking; worry and anxiety impair the lung, but joy conquers worry and anxiety; fear and fright impairs the kidney, but overthinking conquers fear and fright; anger impairs the liver, but sorrow conquers anger. (See Figure 4-1)

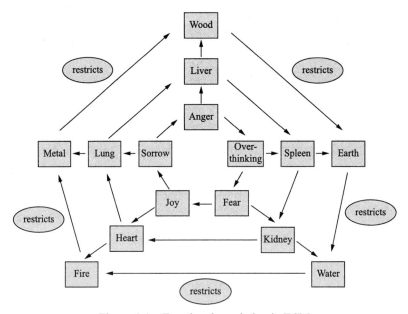

Figure 4-1   Emotional regulation in TCM

You might wonder why it is possible for one emotion to conquer another. It is because emotional change can trigger the change of *qi* activity. *Qi* activity refers to the constant movement of *qi* in the basic forms of ascending, descending, exiting, and entering that maintains various physiological activities of the human body. The changes of *qi* activity may cause disorders. There is a famous saying in 'Fundamental Questions: Pain': 'All diseases originate in *qi* disorders.'

The story of Zhu Danxi treating the female patient is an application of the *qi*-activity theory. Signs and symptoms such as no desire for food or water and depression were caused by excessive thinking, hence *qi* was bound and failed to flow smoothly. To treat it, Zhu Danxi took advantage of the method of using one emotion to conquer another, that is, anger can conquer overthinking. Rage causes *qi* and blood to flow upwards, breaking the knot of *qi* for the time being. To prevent the rebinding of *qi*, the woman was given a letter and told that her husband was coming back soon to make her happy. As a result, her *qi* activity was harmonized, and her mind was unimpeded. She was thus cured.

In ancient times, using one emotion to conquer another was a common therapy for emotion-related disorders. In Chapter 3 of this book, I told you the story that Fan Jin went mad because of his over-joy resulting from his success in the imperial examination. When the surrounding people were at a loss and did not know what to do, the messenger came upon an idea and suggested finding someone that Fan Jin was normally afraid of to threaten him and told him that the news was a fake, that he failed in the imperial examination. His father-in-law, Old Father Hu (胡老爹), a butcher, was asked to do the job. Mr. Hu entered the room, walked up to the poor scholar, whacked him in the mouth and shouted: 'You damn fool. You failed again.' Fan Jin then fainted. When he regained consciousness, his eyes were found bright again and he stopped talking nonsense. He was cured by the method of 'fear conquering joy.'

The method of using one emotion to relieve another is not only used in ancient times but finds its use in modern times. There are a couple of examples of 'using fear to conquer joy' to stave off possible hazards or fatality due to drink driving or over-speeding. In restaurants or on roadside signboards, you won't miss sayings such as 'one drop of wine on the driver's part, two streams of tear on the relatives' part' and 'where there is a good drink there is danger.'

Anger can be conquered by sorrow. When one cries bitterly, one is usually out of breath. According to TCM theory, excessive sorrow exhausts *qi*. As a result, one does not have a feeling as high energy as rage. Hence, anger is relieved.

Q6. How do you vent emotions?

For the sake of health, you are advised to express your feelings and emotions instead of stuffing them inside until you explode one day. Here are a few common methods to release emotional tension, namely, nagging, communication, and exercise.

First, nagging. Nagging can be irritating. But nagging is a way to let out emotions, so nagging should be allowed. As listeners, you should get the point of one's nagging.

My neighbor's wife is a nagging woman. She does chores at home, cleans the floor, cooks meals, and washes dishes. She also works, so she has to do housework after she returns from work. She is exhausted. If she is dissatisfied or feels frustrated, she nags her husband. She often says: 'Look, what if we have a house maid? The maid will do all those chores, and so I don't have to.' Then one day, my neighbor took it seriously. He went to the housekeeping company and hired a maid. When the maid arrived, the lady cried: 'Why did you hire the maid? Did you ask for my opinion?' 'Didn't you say we'd better hire a maid to do the housework?' replied my neighbor. 'Well, I simply vented. How come you took it seriously!' Often, the naggers do not need any feedback at all. They simply want to find somebody who can listen to them.

To cope with nagging, the best strategy is to be a good listener. But remember the old Chinese saying: 'Lend your left ear to what is said and get it out of your right ear.' The ancient Chinese believed that there were three ways of listening. The story is described as follows.

A little wooden figure has two ears and a nose. If a straw is to be inserted from the left ear, there are three possible destinations for the straw. First, the straw is inserted from the left ear and comes out from the right ear. Second, the straw is inserted from the left ear, and nothing comes out. The straw is gone. Third, the straw is inserted from the left ear and comes out of the mouth. What does this story imply? It means there can be three results from listening. One, lend your left ear to what is said and get it out of your right ear. That is, don't take what others say too seriously. Two, listen attentively and keep what you hear in your heart. You hear and you digest. Third, listen attentively and then speak out what you hear. You hear and you spread the message. For a husband, the first strategy is the best option to cope with his wife's nagging. But attention should be paid to the manner of listening. Be sincere and be genuine when you listen.

Second, communication. You should often talk with your friends and family members. You can be very tired after a day's work because almost everyone is under great pressure these days. Communication with your friend or family member is a way of venting your feelings. It is not uncommon for me to treat such patients as the solitary elderly. An increasing number of elderly people are living alone in China nowadays. After their children move out, they have nobody to talk to. For the elderly who live with their children, things are not easy, either. An elderly female patient reported that she didn't want to go out when her children left home for work. She preferred lying in bed and watching TV. More often than not, she would fall asleep during watching. With the passage of time, she became more and more reluctant to communicate with others and was depressed. She thought that life was meaningless and showed no interest in her surroundings. In the end, she fell ill because she felt no desire for food, and she became weak.

For patients like this elderly woman, the best medicine is to communicate with people of their age. Chatting is a way to vent. Indeed, chatting is a way to preserve health.

Third, exercise. If you have ever struggled with frustration or depression, you may have felt much better after you did some sport such as running or playing soccer. Exercise allows a channel for turning your attention and getting something off your chest. The intense emotion is expelled along with your sweat. Activity soothes the flow of *qi* and blood, and your depression is then relieved.

In China, students are required to do exercises during the break. For example, after the first two classes, students and staff usually perform gymnastics on the sportsground according to the broadcast instructions with a tempo. Sinew-transforming Exercise[1] and Eight-section Brocade[2] are also commonly practiced

---

[1] Sinew-transforming Exercise: a form of traditional *qigong* exercise for training tendons and muscles.

[2] Eight-section Brocade: a *qigong* exercise in eight forms, widely practiced by people of all ages in China.

for a break from work. Exercise is a great way to regulate or vent emotions.

Apart from this, psychological consultation centers are available in China where there is an 'anger room.' You can take out your anger there by hitting or smashing the objects in the room: figures, a bed, cups made of cotton flannel, sandbags and even rubber dummies, if you'd like. In other parts of the world, there are sport centers specialized in helping people vent their aggressive impulses. Those in need of venting can smash anything or shout out loud in the room. I once had the chance to visit one of those rooms. There was a TV set equipped with a tennis game software. You can play tennis with someone appearing on the TV screen. After playing for some time, you will have your attention focused on hitting tennis balls and your negative emotion can be mitigated.

Therefore, physical activity and sports provide a platform for people to release their tension. Emotional ventilation is a therapy that is also emphasized in *Huangdi's Inner Canon of Medicine*. According to 'Fundamental Questions: Significant Discussions on the Changing Principles of Six *Qi*' (*Sù Wèn Liù Yuán Zhèng Jì Dà Lùn* 素问•六元正纪大论), 'When liver (wood) *qi* has stagnated, smooth its way; when heart (fire) *qi* has stagnated, disperse it; when spleen (earth) *qi* has stagnated, resolve it; when lung (metal) *qi* has stagnated, drain it; when kidney (water) *qi* has stagnated, inhibit it.'

Based on the above quote, disorders such as oppression or depression can be relieved through opening a channel. This is what TCM emphasizes for the treatment of diseases. When pathogenic *qi* invades the human body, the wisest alternative is to drive it out. When *qi* or blood has stagnated and you feel distressful or depressed, it is better to find an outlet for your negative emotions.

Q7. What does it mean that nourishing the spirit is to nourish the body?

The heart governs the spirit. Through regulating your mindset and emotions and performing emotional ventilation, you can maintain your mind-body health and spiritual wellbeing. The heart spirit is believed to govern both physical and mental activities. When there is spiritual wellness, there will be physical wellbeing. This is what *Huangdi's Inner Canon of Medicine* aims to say: nourishing your spirit is to nourish your physical wellbeing.

Searching for fun in everyday life is part of the ideas in the opening chapter of the *Canon*. For instance, according to 'Fundamental Questions: Genuine *Qi* Endowed by Heaven in Remote Antiquity,' you should 'consider your food delicious, accept your clothes, and enjoy folk custom.' If you are content with what you have, with no personal considerations, you will 'attain a tranquil mind and you are without fear of anything.' In this case, 'no desire or want can tempt your eyes; no obscenity or evil can confuse your mind.' That is, you won't be tempted by any excessiveness or bad things in the outside world. You can 'obtain both spiritual and physical wellness, fulfill the allotted span, and live to be more than a hundred years old.'

Chapter 5
The Secret to Heart Fire

Q1. Why does the heart pertain to fire?

In summer, we prefer cold dishes or salads pleasant to the palate. A lot of us would eat watermelon to cool down and stay hydrated. According to TCM, eating these food and fruits can reduce heart fire or prevent it from being in excess. Summer corresponds to fire as is described by the theory of five elements. But why does the heart pertain to fire?

There are two reasons. First, color associations. Chinese understanding of anatomy can be found in *Huangdi's Inner Canon of Medicine*. For instance, some discourses in *Miraculous Pivot* such as 'The Relationship Between Rivers and Channels' and 'Intestines and the Stomach' describe the length of digestive system and specific data regarding diameter is given to the esophagus, the stomach, the small and large intestines. By dissecting bodies, the ancient Chinese found that the heart was mainly red, and it stored blood. The blood was red, too. In ancient times, red was associated with fire. Hence, the heart is related to fire.

The other important factor that contributes to this relationship is the power of the heart. The heart beats and pumps blood throughout the human body to sustain life. From the perspective of the five elements, fire is the most powerful one. That's why the heart is associated with fire.

Do you remember the saying that the heart governs *shen* (神, spirit)? *Shen* is related to the heart. The ancient Chinese also believe that '*shen* is the essence of fire.' If something is changeable, unpredictable, and capable of doing what is beyond man's imagination, it is called *shen* (magic). A magic doctor, therefore, is a highly skilled doctor who can relieve a disorder that no one believes there is a cure for it. In terms of the five elements, fire flickers and its shape may constantly change. Hence, fire is related to *shen*.

To sum up, the heart pertains to fire in terms of the five elements and it governs *shen* (spirit).

Q2. What are the two aspects of the heart being related to fire?

The notion that the heart is related to fire can be expounded from the following two aspects: insufficiency and excess of heart fire. Questions 3–4 provide more details.

Q3. What is insufficiency of heart fire?

Insufficiency of heart fire can also be called insufficiency of heart *yang*. Its signs and symptoms include but are not limited to pain or tightness in the chest, shortness of breath, purplish lips, and bluish-greenish complexion. It can be angina if chest pain is the main symptom. In addition to pectoral pain, some patients may have a feeling of suffocation and tend to take deep breaths, which is called frequent sighing. These are attributed to insufficient heart fire. This pattern of disharmony is called chest *bi* (痹) or chest impediment in TCM. *Bi* means obstruction or impediment. That is, the flow of heart *qi* is impeded. As a result, there is a feeling of oppression. Sometimes the back aches, the lips are purplish, and the complexion can be bluish-greenish. To treat it, Cassia Twig and Licorice Decoction (*Guì Zhī Gān Cǎo Tāng* 桂枝甘草汤) is commonly used. As the name suggests, it contains only two ingredients.

Cassia Twig (*guì zhī* 桂枝) tastes pungent and somewhat sweet and is warm in property. It enters the heart meridian and is used to boost *yang qi* of the heart to enable a forceful heartbeat. Licorice (*gān cǎo* 甘草) is a guide ingredient which can direct medicinal action to the affected meridian. It harmonizes the ingredients and can direct action to the twelve principal meridians of the whole body. Licorice replenishes *qi* and tonifies the heart. This herbal decoction is used for patients with palpitations, tightness in the chest, and pain.

In severe cases characterized by a feeling of suffocation, profuse phlegm, chest tightness, and pain accompanied with backache, use Decoction of Snakegourd Fruit, Longstamen Onion and *Bai Jiu* (*Guā Lóu Xiè Bái Bái Jiǔ Tāng* 瓜蔞薤白白 酒汤). Snakegourd Fruit (*guā lóu* 瓜蔞) regulates *qi*, soothes the chest, resolves phlegm, and opens the channel for *qi* to flow. Longstamen Onion (*xiè bái* 薤白), pungent in taste and warm in property, is used to improve heart function. It regulates *yang qi* of the heart and removes stagnation. Zhang Zhongjing of the Eastern Han dynasty combined the use of Snakegourd Fruit and Longstamen Onion together for the treatment of many diseases. *Bai Jiu* (白酒 , Chinese distilled spirits or Chinese liquor) is pungent and warm. If you drink some, you will feel warm. For some people, their face will be flushed, or their complexion will turn red after drinking. According to *Huangdi's Inner Canon of Medicine*, in remote antiquity, spirits were prepared but not consumed because people at that time emphasized nurturing life and they rarely fell ill. That is, only if people occasionally got sick and needed them for medical treatment would they be put into use. So, in ancient times, spirits were used as medicinal ingredients. Consider the traditional Chinese character for medicine (*yī* 醫). You will find that it is made of the upper character 殹 (*yī* medicine) and the lower character 酉 (*yǒu* liquor). The upper character is used as a phonetic and the lower character is a pictograph of a wine cask.

In middle antiquity, morality declined. People sought fame and became materialistic. With decreased healthy *qi*, they were more susceptible to the invasion of pathogenic factors. But taking some liquor could still help them restore health. Then Huangdi asked why people at the present time couldn't get cured by taking some liquor. According to 'Fundamental Questions: Soups and Liquors' (*Sù Wèn Tāng Yè Láo Lǐ Lùn* 素问·汤液醪醴论), Qibo replied that people nowadays had to take herbal decoction to relieve internal disorders and to use needles and moxa to treat external diseases. In the original text, the expression '*du yao*' (毒 药 , literally toxic medicine) is used. Nevertheless, the Chinese character 毒 does not mean toxin or toxic as what is understood today. It carries a specific meaning here, referring to the medicinal properties that are peculiar to an herbal ingredient. It is believed that the combined use of liquor and other herbs with their medicinal properties can contribute to the removal of disorders.

Liquor is pungent in taste and warm in property and therefore is used to raise up the spirit. The ancient Chinese call liquor 'cooked grain product,' that is, liquor is produced when grains are brewed and fermented. There is a phenomenon: the urine transformed from liquor is discharged before food is digested. 'Miraculous Pivot: Generation and Convergence of Nutrient *Qi* and Defense *Qi*' (*Líng Shū Yíng Wèi Shēng Huì* 灵枢•营卫生会) reads: 'Liquor is taken into the stomach after food but is discharged before food is digested.' This is the effect of liquor on the human body. It produces urine flow, warms you, and makes your face flushed. Pungent in taste and warm and mobile in property, liquor can be used to treat coronary heart diseases caused by insufficiency of heart fire.

When heart fire is insufficient, the function of the heart will be affected. Then coronary heart disease or myocardial infarction may occur. Some patients can be characterized by dyspnea. They are unable to lie down and have to lean against something. When heart failure occurs, the heart is unable to pump blood around the human body efficiently. Then the patient may present symptoms such as swelling in the abdomen and sometimes pulmonary edema.

The incidence rate is relatively high for coronary heart diseases or what we call chest impediment including myocardial infarction. Nowadays, it could be listed in the top three of the incidence rate or mortality rate. Several of my friends died of myocardial infarction with very urgent and sudden onset. Thus, caution should be exercised.

Q4. What is excess of heart fire?

Excess of heart fire means heart *yang* is in excess. In clinical practice, it is common to see patients whose signs and symptoms are characterized by restlessness, red face, red tongue, sores on the mouth and tongue, erosion on the tip of the tongue, and yellow urine. Several factors contribute to the excess of heart fire. Diet, for example, is one of the causes. If you eat too much chili and other foods of hot property, you might have an excess of heart fire. A man told me that he craved for lychee. He lives in the northern part of China and used to eat few lichees. But one day, he went to Guangzhou (in the southern part of China) on a business trip and happened to eat some lychees. He found that they were delicious with sweet juicy white flesh. Then he bought one kilogram and ate them all. On the following day, he had sores on his mouth and tongue and even nosebleeds. As you can see, improper diet may cause excess of heart fire.

Other than this, the six climatic factors such as wind, cold, summer-heat, dampness, dryness, and fire can transform into pathogenic fire when they become excessive.

Furthermore, *qi* depression transforms into fire. It is said that desires minus capabilities equals inflammation or fire. That is, if your ability is not great enough to meet your desires or wants, you will feel stressed and depressed. If depression persists, it will transform into fire. In terms of TCM, *qi* in excess turns into fire. In clinical practice, examining the tongue will help diagnose and determine hear fire. In cases of excessive heart fire, signs and symptoms include a red tongue, especially redness in the tip of the tongue and sores on mouth and tongue.

Q5. What does your tongue say about your heart health?

According to *Huangdi's Inner Canon of Medicine*, each of the five sensory organs is paired with one of the five *zang*-organs that eyes with the liver, nose with the lung, ears with the kidney, mouth with the spleen, and tongue with the heart. 'Fundamental Questions: Significant Discussions on Phenomena Corresponding to *Yin* and *Yang*' (*Sù Wèn Yīn Yáng Yìng Xiàng Dà Lùn* 素问·阴阳应象大论) reads: 'The heart rules the tongue... The tongue is the window of the heart.' That is, the heart condition is usually manifested in the tongue. But why is it? There are two reasons.

First, the ancient Chinese believed that the collateral of the Heart Meridian of Hand Lesser *Yin* was connected to the root of the tongue.

Second, it is based on observation and clinical experience. When you have mental restlessness, chances are that you have a red tongue. When the tip of your tongue is red and there is erosion on its surface, medicinals for removing heart fire work effectively. Over time, ancients concluded that the heart rules the tongue.

Some people may wonder why the original text states that the tongue is a *qiao* (窍 , orifice or opening) similar to the other sensory organs such as eyes, nose, mouth, and ears. The tongue is not an opening. Why would the text say, 'the heart opens to the tongue'? Actually, the character 窍 has three different meanings. The first meaning is run-through. As 'Miraculous Pivot: Length of Meridians' (*Líng Shū Mài Dù* 灵枢·脉度) reads: 'Heart *qi* flows to the tongue. Only when the heart is in harmony can the tongue recognize the five flavors[①].' The second meaning is key or pivot. It makes sense when we say the tongue is pivotal to the examination of the heart's condition. The third meaning is opening. We could say that the tongue has openings because there are taste buds on the tongue so that we can enjoy the flavors. All sense organs in fact have openings to perceive what is outside. Take the skin, for example. There are sweat pores. In TCM, sweat pores are called *xuan fu* (玄府 , literally mysterious residence). One of the meanings of the character *xuan* (玄) is 'water' because it is the place where water is stored. Another meaning is 'mystery' because the opening is too minute to be seen. Sweat pores are also called *qi men* (气 门 , literally the door of *qi*), meaning that they are the openings or passages for the dispersion of *qi*.

Q6. What is the clinical significance of the heart ruling the tongue?

The heart rules the tongue; that is, the tongue is the external manifestation of the heart condition. The tongue is related to taste and speech. Its function depends

---

① five flavors: referring to various tastes such as sweet, sour, bitter, pungent, and salty.

on the physiological functions of the heart such as governing blood, vessels, and the mind. Because no epidermis covers the tongue and its blood vessels are abundant, it is easy to detect by observing the color and luster of the tongue and by examining the circulation of *qi* and blood and the physiological function of the heart governing blood and vessels. If the heart functions normally, the tongue will be healthily red, lustrous, soft, and flexible with acute sense of taste. Speech is fluent. If the heart is diseased, it can be reflected on the tongue. For example, a red tip and erosion on the tongue indicate excess of heart fire. A pale tongue and white greasy coating indicate insufficiency of heart *qi*. In addition, pathological changes of taste, a stiff tongue, and sluggish speech may occur.

In clinical practice, I once had a patient with sequela of a cerebrovascular disease. He complained that everything he ate tasted the same flavor of spiced peanuts, whether it was a fried long bean, bean sprouts, or braised pork. He felt very miserable and lost his appetite. This made him think that life was boring. The cause of this disease was heart *qi* failing to reach the tongue; hence, the tongue lost its tasting ability. I treated him by harmonizing his heart *qi*. When his heart *qi* was regulated, his taste perception gradually recovered. After several rounds of treatment, he was cured. He said that he was able to taste the delicious braised pork and differentiate other flavors such as spicy, sour, and so on. This is an application of the concept that 'heart *qi* flows to the tongue and only when the heart is in harmony can the tongue recognize the five flavors.'

Q7. What does your urine say about your heart health?

Your urine can also tell you about your heart health. If someone reports that they have yellow urine and difficult or painful urination, a Western medicine doctor may say it is a urinary tract infection whereas a TCM doctor characterizes it as 'small intestinal fire.' This kind of patients usually has signs and symptoms such as having a red tongue, oral sores, and mental restlessness. Redness-removing Powder (*Dǎo Chì Sǎn* 导赤散) is usually used to clear heart heat and induce diuresis. It contains four ingredients, namely, Unprocessed Rehmannia Root (*shēng dì* 生地),

Tip of Licorice Root (*gān cǎo shāo* 甘草梢), Lophatherum Herb (*zhú yè* 竹叶), and Armand Clematis Stem (*chuān mù tōng* 川木通). The therapy is used in accordance with the TCM belief that a *zang*-organ is often paired with a *fu*-organ, forming an interior-exterior relationship. For the heart, it is paired with the small intestine. Thus, heart fire can be reduced by promoting urination.

Perhaps it is easier to understand that the liver is paired with the gallbladder, the spleen with the stomach, the kidney with the bladder because they are close to one another. But for the heart with the small intestine and the lung with the large intestine, they seem to be distant in location from one another. How can they be paired? It is because each of the collaterals of *zang*-organs is connected to a particular *fu*-organ. The meridians of *zang*-organs are *yin* and those of *fu*-organs are *yang*. Each *yin* meridian is paired with a *yang* meridian. For example, the Heart Meridian of Hand Lesser *Yin* connects to the Small Intestine of Hand Greater *Yang* at the little finger. (See Figure 5-1 and Figure 5-2)

Yin meridians: connected with the five *zang*-organs

Three *yin* meridians of the hand: on the inner side of the upper limbs
- Lung Meridian of Hand Greater *Yin*
- Pericardium Meridian of Hand Reverting *Yin*
- Heart Meridian of Hand Lesser *Yin*

Three *yin* meridians of the foot: on the inner side of the lower limbs
- Spleen Meridian of Foot Greater *Yin*
- Liver Meridian of Foot Reverting *Yin*
- Kidney Meridian of Foot Lesser *Yin*

Figure 5-1   Classification of *yin* meridians

Yang meridians: connected with the six *fu*-organs

Three *yang* meridians of the hand: on the outer side of the upper limbs
- Large Intestine Meridian of Hand *Yang* Brightness
- Triple Energizer Meridian of Hand Lesser *Yang*
- Small Intestine Meridian of Hand Greater *Yang*

Three *yang* meridians of the foot: on the outer side of the lower limbs
- Stomach Meridian of Foot *Yang* Brightness
- Gallbladder Meridian of Foot Lesser *Yang*
- Bladder Meridian of Foot Greater *Yang*

Figure 5-2   Classification of *yang* meridians

Furthermore, clinical experience proves that the heart and the small intestine affect each other pathologically. When there is fire in the heart meridian, it can transfer heat to the small intestine, which causes symptoms like oliguria, reddish urine, and stabbing pain. Those with urinary problems such as difficulty or pain in urination often show the signs and symptoms of excessive heart fire. In addition, the therapy of promoting diuresis is often found effective for relieving heart fire. Thanks to this accumulated experience, it is believed that the heart and the small intestine are related, and their meridians are of interior-exterior relationship.

Perhaps you will argue that the urine is released from the bladder, not the small intestine. According to the Canon, the bladder is where fluids are stored, and the small intestine is where transformation takes place. The small intestine transforms things, separates purified nutrients from turbid wastes and absorbs nutrients of food and drinks as well as water and fluids. The purified nutrients are transformed through spleen *qi* into blood to nourish the heart and vessels. The solid and formed wastes are then removed out of the body from the large intestine while waste liquids are released from the bladder. Therefore, the small intestine is paired with the heart.

Q8. Why does the heart manifest its splendor in the face?

'Miraculous Pivot: Symptoms of *Zang-fu* Organs Due to the Invasion of Pathogenic *Qi*' states: 'Humans have twelve meridians and three hundred and sixty-five collaterals. Their *qi* and blood all flow into the face and infuse into its orifices.' The *qi* and blood in the meridians are controlled by the heart, so the heart manifests its splendor in the face. That is, the face can mirror the condition of the heart.

We all have such an experience in winter. When winter hits the street, a great many of us will wear hats, gloves, and coats. Some of us may also wear masks to protect the nose and the mouth because the air outside is cold and perhaps dirty. For ears, we have earmuffs to protect from cold. In other words, all parts of the body except for the face are covered. The face seems to be more resistant to cold. Why is it? It is because the *qi* and blood of the twelve meridians and three hundred and sixty-five collaterals all flow into the face. The heart governs blood and vessels and pertains to fire. Therefore, the heart rules the face, and the face is more resistant to cold. In clinical practice, pale complexion indicates insufficiency of heart blood. Red face and eyes indicate the excess of heart fire. Bluish-greenish facial complexion and purplish lips indicate blood stagnation. As is described, the condition of the heart can be mirrored in the face.

Q9. What does it mean that the face is a miniature of the human body?

Though the face overall is ruled by the heart, each part of it, according to the Canon, can be specially related to a specific part of the human body. That is, the face is a miniature of the human body. For example, the forehead is related to the head. The part between the forehead and the eyebrows is related to the throat. The midpoint between the eyebrows called ophryon is ruled by the lung. The root of the nose between the eyes is ruled by the heart. The nose bridge is ruled by the liver. The two sides of the nose bridge are ruled by the gallbladder, and the nose-guard is ruled by the spleen. The wings of the nose are ruled by the stomach. The parts below the cheekbones are ruled by the large intestine. The sides of the parts below the cheekbones are ruled by the kidney. The philtrum is ruled by the bladder and the uterus. In sum, each part of the face pertains to a specific organ. This is another theory put forward in *Huangdi's Inner Canon of Medicine*, which can be called the extension of the theory of five elements storing each other[1].

Q10. Why is the heart related to the *qi* of summer?

The heart is in the upper part of the body and pertains to *yang*. Besides, the heart beats and pumps blood and pertains to fire. Hence, it is the greater *yang* of *yang*. TCM considers man and nature to be a unity. Each of the five seasons is

---

[1] the five elements storing each other: each of the five elements can be subdivided into five elements.

believed to correspond to an element and a *zang*-organ and/or *fu*-organ. For example, spring corresponds to the element of wood and the liver; summer to the element of fire and the heart; late summer to the element of earth and the spleen-stomach; autumn to the element of metal and the lung; and winter to the element of water and the kidney. That is why 'Fundamental Questions: Six-Plus-Six System and the Manifestations of the Viscera' states that the heart is related to the *qi* of summer.

Q11. Why are you prone to air-conditioning disease in summer?

In summer, you may like to eat cold dishes and watermelons to relieve summer heat. Some of you also like to stay in an air-conditioned room. Over time, there arises a disorder called air-conditioning disease. If you stay in an air-conditioned room for a long time in summer, you may have an aversion to cold, weak limbs, and a poor appetite. Some may also have headaches, backaches, and limb pain. This is the result of inappropriate use of air conditioning. The cause is that you seldom go outdoors and have less exposure to sunshine. Then the *yang qi* in your body cannot be released. In fact, in summertime the temperatures rage. Meanwhile, the human body is governed by the heart and the heart pertains to fire. Your sweat pores are open and muscular interstices are flabby. The *yang qi* of the human body can exit the body in the form of sweat. Because sweating can regulate your body temperature, it will prevent you from having excessive heart fire. Therefore, moderate sweating is good for you in summer.

However, some people prefer staying in an air-conditioned room without going outdoors. On one hand, cold air can invade the human body through opened sweat pores. On the other hand, according to TCM, cold rules contraction, so cold air makes sweat pores close off. As a result, *yang qi* is blocked in the body and cannot go out, which causes the absence of sweating. In this case, there is cold on the exterior and heat enclosed in the interior, developing a pattern of disharmony called 'cold enveloping fire,' the so-called air-conditioning disease, characterized by headaches, fever, aversion to cold, absence of sweating, pain in the limbs and even vomiting and diarrhea.

Q12. How do you preserve health in summer?

There are four ways for you to preserve health in summer so that you retain your fire energy without making it excessive.

First, increase activity to allow the release of *yang qi*.

'Fundamental Questions: Significant Discussions on Regulating the Spirit in Accordance with the *Qi* of the Four Seasons' (*Sù Wèn Sì Qì Tiáo Shén Dà Lùn* 四气调神大论) states: 'The three months of summer denote exuberance and picturesque scenery. The *qi* of heaven (*yang*) and earth (*yin*) interact, and myriad things bloom and bear fruit.' To accommodate the environment, people should 'go to rest late at night and rise early. Do not detest the long daytime or complain about the hot weather.' The top priority of the things you should do in summer is to increase your activity and take up some outdoor activities instead of staying in an air-conditioned room.

Second, keep energetic without getting angry.

The text goes on to say: 'Keep a good mood and avoid anger. Make yourself as energetic as the full-blossomed trees and green grass in nature. Cause the *qi* to flow away, as if what you loved were located outside.' As is known to all, anger won't be generated for no reason. It usually comes with depression. One may feel depressed upon hearing something unpleasant. When the depression reaches a certain level, it will blow up and turn into fury. So, in my opinion, to avoid anger doesn't mean that you don't release your distress at all. Rather, you try to avoid getting depressed. How can you do that? My advice is to let out what you feel or think. In other words, speak exactly what is on your mind instead of brooding over it if you do have a strong reaction to it. To put it another way, in summertime, you tend to have a stronger capacity for reaction and are apt to be more straight-forward. This is also the indication of *yang* ruling the exterior. Therefore, you are not advised to hold in until it blows up. In fact, cultivating health in summer is about how you nourish your heart.

Third, prevent heatstroke.

It is not wise for you to directly bask in the hot sun for a long time in the summer. Otherwise, you may collapse.

According to 'Fundamental Questions: Significant Discussions on Regulating the Spirit in Accordance with the *Qi* of the Four Seasons,' 'cause the *qi* to flow away, as if that what you loved were located outside. This brings into correspondence with the *qi* of summer and is the principle for health preservation. Opposing it impairs the heart.' Summertime tends to have excessive heat. You are advised to work up a sweat to release some *yang qi* in your body. Hence, moderate outdoor activities are necessary for health preservation. If this principle is violated, heart *qi* can be impaired.

Nevertheless, 'Fundamental Questions: Change of Essence and Transformation of *Qi*' warns you that you should 'stay in the shade to avoid summer-heat.' Proper care should be taken not to be exposed to direct sunlight. When it is too hot, it is better for you to cool down to prevent the excess of heart fire. Here, it does not mean that you stay in an air-conditioned room for a long time. You can have a temporary stay for regulation to avoid excessive summer heat. Please keep in mind that moderation is of critical importance. Sun Simiao (孙思邈)[1] put forward three rules for health preservation in summer: 'Don't be greedy for coolness and shade; don't sleep under the stars and the moon; and don't use a fan during sleep.' That is, you should not stay in a cool place for too long. You shouldn't sleep in an open field or under a big tree. At night, when you sleep you shouldn't keep the electric fan or the air conditioner on all the time. Otherwise, you will likely catch a cold. Therefore, relaxation in the shade should be done in moderation.

Apart from this, moderate eating is also of vital importance for health preservation. In summertime, the purpose of eating cold dishes and watermelon is to prevent the excess of heart fire. Watermelon is called natural White Tiger Decoction (*Bái Hǔ Tāng* 白虎汤) by the ancient Chinese. Because watermelon is sweet and juicy, it can clear away heat, generate fluids and prevent heatstroke. It is called natural White Tiger Decoction because White Tiger Decoction is a classic herbal formula of Zhang Zhongjing to remove high fever. White tiger is the divine beast of the west which represents the autumn dryness of the west. When the *qi* of autumn dryness arrives, the *qi* of summer heat disappears. Therefore, White Tiger Decoction

---

① Sun Simiao (孙思邈): a well-known Chinese physician of the Tang dynasty and the author of the *Prescriptions Worth a Thousand Pieces of Gold* (*Qiān Jīn Fāng* 千金方).

is used to treat patients with intense fever. Eating watermelons, the natural decoction, in summer is good for you to cool down and produce fluids to prevent heatstroke. Of course, caution should be taken. Keep in mind that moderation is crucial: excessive consumption may harm your body.

Fourth, cultivate *yang* in summertime.

Yang qi in nature reaches the highest level in summer. So does the *yang qi* in the human body. For people with insufficiency of *yang qi*, it is appropriate to replenish *yang qi* in summertime. 'Fundamental Questions: Significant Discussions on Regulating the Spirit in Accordance with the *Qi* of the Four Seasons' states: 'Cultivate *yang* in spring and summer.' Several diseases are common in winter, for instance, tracheitis, bronchial asthma, and some rheumatic diseases. In winter, patients with rheumatoid arthritis will usually find their condition aggravated. Some TCM physicians ascribe it to the *yang* deficiency of the spleen, the kidney, and the heart. Since summer is the season with relatively hot weather and the human body has sufficient *yang*, it is an efficient way to supplement *yang* at this time of the year. That is why TCM physicians recommend treating winter diseases in summer. This is part of the strategy of preventive medicine.

One more thing is worthy of attention. In summer some patients with *yang* deficiency are likely to have diarrhea, loss of appetite, and vomiting. In this case, their *yang qi* should be replenished. Medical consultation should be obtained promptly.

Chapter 6
General's Power

Q1. What does TCM say about the liver's function?

When liver *qi* becomes hyperactive and there is fire generated internally, patients are irritable and tend to lose temper easily. Such patients often ask TCM doctors whether they should have a liver-function test. Actually, the liver in TCM is somewhat different from that in Western medicine.

According to Western medicine, liver is involved with metabolism of protein, fat, and carbohydrate, and also has the functions of detoxification, hematopoiesis, and coagulation.

The liver's function in TCM needs to be interpreted from the formation of the Chinese character 肝 (*gān*, liver). According to *Brightness Hall Discourse on the Five Zang-Organs* (*Míng Táng Wǔ Zàng Lùn* 明堂五脏论), a surviving volume of an ancient medical book in Dunhuang in the province of Gansu, 肝 means 干 (*gān*). *Er Ya* (*Ěr Yǎ* 尔雅), a monograph on the meaning of Chinese characters and words, explains the character 干 as 扞 (*hàn*), which indicates that the liver has the function of defending and guarding.

There is a saying in 'Fundamental Questions: Secret Canon Stored in the Royal

Library': 'The liver functions as a general and strategic thinking originates from there.' As is known to us, generals are in charge of national defense, and they will mobilize their troops to defend the country whenever the enemy invades. In the human body, the liver plays the role of an army general, and its troop is what TCM calls *qi*. The liver's mobilization of *qi* is mainly manifested in its regulation of blood circulation, emotional and spiritual activities, digestive function, and reproductive function. Only when liver *qi* flows freely can the above four aspects be in a normal state. Therefore, the liver's function in TCM can be summarized as 'the liver governing coursing and discharge.'

Q2. What are the characteristics of *qi*?

There are three characteristics of *qi*. First, *qi* is not entirely functional; it is corporeal. Although *qi* is intangible, it is indeed a substance with energy. It is mentioned in *Huangdi's Inner Canon of Medicine* that when *qi* accumulates, substance is formed. The formed substance here makes *qi* visible and tangible. Second, *qi* is not static, but in motion. *Qi* is moving and ubiquitous, and it can flow anywhere in the universe. Third, *qi* is perceptible. Although *qi* is invisible and intangible, it can be perceived through its signs and manifestations.

Q3. What is the relationship between *qi* and blood?

Qi and blood are seemingly two different substances. *Qi* is invisible and pertains to *yang*, while blood is a red liquid and pertains to *yin*. In fact, *qi* and blood are closely related. TCM thinks that '*qi* is the commander of blood,' which means blood follows the movement of *qi*, or *qi* drives the movement of blood. The mobilization of *qi* can be perceived from the direction of blood flow.

There are often such scenes in TV dramas: when someone bursts into a rage, they feel dizzy, cover their chest with hands, and then fall to the ground unconscious. 'Fundamental Questions: The Interrelationship between Life and Nature' (*Sù Wèn*

Shēng Qì Tōng Tiān Lùn 素问·生气通天论) explains this as: 'Rage drives *qi* to move upward, upsetting the harmony of the physical body. Blood rushes upwards and stagnates in the head, leading to syncope.' In other words, for people with great anger, their liver will mobilize *qi* and blood excessively, affecting their heart and brain, resulting in their sudden unconsciousness.

The Romance of the Three Kingdoms (*Sān Guó Yǎn Yì* 三国演义) tells a story. After the victory of the Battle of Red Cliff (赤壁之战)[1], both Sun Quan (孙权) and Liu Bei (刘备) wanted to occupy Jingzhou (荆州)[2] where the troops of Cao Cao (曹操) had been stationed. Sun Quan's army arrived first, but they failed to capture Jingzhou in their first attack because of their underestimation of the opponent. Zhou Yu (周瑜), Sun Quan's military counsellor, then formulated a plan to trick Cao Cao's army out and attacked them again. However, when they defeated Cao Cao, they were astonished to find that Jingzhou had been occupied by Guan Yu (关羽), Liu Bei's sworn brother. To get Jingzhou back, Zhou Yu made another plan to ask Sun Shangxiang (孙尚香), Sun Quan's sister, to pretend to marry Liu Bei, so that Liu Bei would be summoned from Jingzhou to Dongwu (东吴)[3]. Zhou Yu intended to detain Liu Bei in Dongwu and asked Zhuge Liang (诸葛亮), Liu Bei's military counsellor, to exchange him for Jingzhou. Unfortunately, his plan was sabotaged by Zhuge Liang's three tips in the embroidered pouches which were given to Zhao Yun (赵云), a general who accompanied Liu Bei to Dongwu. Eventually, Liu Bei married Sun Shangxiang successfully, and Zhou Yu's army was ambushed by Zhuge Liang's when they were chasing Liu Bei. What made Zhou Yu more ashamed was that Zhuge Liang then asked his soldiers to shout all over the street that 'Zhou's brilliant plan of conquest has cost him the lady and the troops.' After a series of failures and humiliations, Zhou Yu was so angry that the arrow wounds he had suffered in the previous battles recurred, and he vomited blood and fainted to the ground. Thus, it is evident that rage causes *qi* and blood to move upward and even leads to vomiting blood and fainting.

---

[1] Battle of Red Cliff (赤壁之战): a battle at the end of the Eastern Han dynasty in 208, in which Liu Bei and Sun Quan jointly crushed Cao Cao.

[2] Jingzhou (荆州): a city in the present Hubei province, China.

[3] Dongwu (东吴): a city now called Suzhou in Jiangsu province, China.

Sometimes, however, physicians can make use of rage to treat diseases. Since rage can stimulate the liver to move *qi* and blood, the method of infuriating patients can be used to treat the diseases caused by *qi* stagnation or blood stasis. A story related to this method can be found in *Records of the Three Kingdoms* (*Sān Guó Zhì* 三国志). There was a prefecture chief who was honest and upright and was loved by the people. Due to overwork, he had suffered from *qi* and blood stagnation for a long time. He consulted many doctors and tried a variety of treatments, but nothing worked. One day, Hua Tuo (华佗), a famous doctor at the time, came to the chief's home and asked to stay there for a few days. Feeling honored and hoping the disease can be cured, the chief agreed to the request and treated Hua Tuo with a great dinner. At the dinner table, the chief seriously described his illness, but Hua Tuo didn't seem to care about it and kept talking anything but his illness. When the dinner was almost finished, Hua Tuo said: 'Though physicians are supposed to save the dying and heal the wounded, they have to make a living anyway.' The chief understood what Hua meant and gave him a big sum of money. Afterwards, Hua Tuo felt the pulse of the chief and did nothing more. No prescription! No Needling! Before returning to his room, he said to the chief: 'Your disease is a bit complicated. Let's wait until tomorrow.' The following day, Hua Tuo repeated what he said and didn't prescribe any medicine to the chief. One day after another, the chief heard the same words and got no treatment. A few days later, the chief was impatient and went to see Hua Tuo, but he found that Hua Tuo had left, leaving only a farewell letter. Hua Tuo said in his letter that he did not want to treat the chief at all, so it was not appropriate for him to stay for free food and drinks. He also wrote that the money given to him was nothing compared with what had been plundered by the chief from the folk people, so he took it away. After reading the letter, the chief flew into a rage, vomited some black blood, and fainted to the ground. When he woke up, he found his son, who had been away for a long time, was about to give him some medicine. His son told the chief that it was he who invited Hua Tuo over, and what had happened was part of the treatment aiming to infuriate the chief and eliminate blood stasis from his body. After that, the chief's condition gradually improved and finally he restored his health.

Q4. How does the liver regulate *qi* and blood?

After a heavy meal, most people would prefer to sit or lie down to rest rather than move about. This is because blood flows to the spleen and stomach to help with digestion while the rest of the body is weak due to the lack of blood. Likewise, when one is occupied with study and thinking, more blood will flow to the heart and the brain; when one is walking, more blood flows to the legs. Such blood flow and circulation are regulated by the liver. As is stated in 'Fundamental Questions: Various Relationships of the Five *Zang*-Organs' (*Sù Wèn Wǔ Zàng Shēng Chéng Piān* 素问•五脏生成篇), 'when the liver receives blood, one can see; when the feet receive blood, one can walk; when the palms receive blood, one can grasp; when the fingers receive blood, one can hold.'

The liver is likened to the army general, who can mobilize *qi* of the body. And *qi* will guide the blood to the organs and tissues that need it. TCM physicians believe that someone who is deficient in *qi* and blood needs to have them replenished, which shows that *qi* and blood are closely related and are often mentioned together. During the day, *qi* and blood move to where they are needed, and at night 'blood returns to the liver when one lies down,' as is described in 'Fundamental Questions: Various Relationships of the Five *Zang*-Organs.' Only by providing enough rest for *qi* and blood can they better carry out their next day's work and help people maintain health.

Moreover, regulated by the liver, *qi* and blood are also gathered in the diseased part of the body. The amount of *qi* and blood that accumulates in the affected area reflects the strength of healthy *qi* in the human body. When one falls ill, their healthy *qi* will fight back and try to remove pathogenic *qi*. Therefore, where there is pathogenic *qi*, there is healthy *qi* to battle it. In other words, *qi* and blood are mostly gathered in the diseased part to support healthy *qi* to restore health. For example, TCM doctors often say that one has a floating pulse when one has a cold. This means that the pulse can be felt by applying light fingertip pressure but grow faint on hard pressure, much like wood floating on water. The rationale of floating pulse is related to the gathering of *qi* and blood on the body surface. TCM believes that colds are often caused by external pathogens invading the body surface and that the liver is responsible for mobilizing *qi* and blood to fight against those pathogens. With a large amount of *qi* and blood distributed on the body surface, the pulse will present a floating state. One is advised to rest more and work less when having a cold, to protect one's *qi* and blood as soon as possible from being consumed to drive away pathogenic *qi*.

Q5. How does the liver regulate emotional activities?

The liver in TCM is closely related to emotions. It is generally acknowledged that generals are always resolute and of a strong temper. They are good at fighting and are thoughtful and resourceful when they fight. The liver is compared to a general. As 'Fundamental Questions: Secret Canon Stored in the Royal Library' states: 'The liver functions as a general and strategic thinking originates from there.' It can be observed in daily life that those who are easily angry seldom have good strategies. Only when one is calm can one think rationally and wisely. That is, the liver functions on the premise of normal emotional activities. Moreover, normal emotional activities depend on the free flow of *qi* and blood. The smooth mobilization of *qi* by the liver in return ensures a calm mood.

Malfunction of the liver will lead to abnormal emotional activities. 'Miraculous Pivot: Basic State of Spirit' states: 'Deficiency of liver *qi* causes fear whereas excess of liver *qi* causes anger.' When *qi* and blood are excessively mobilized by the liver, liver fire will be generated, and people are likely to become furious. When *qi* and blood are mobilized too little by the liver, liver *qi* will become stagnant, and people are likely to get depressed.

Depression is a very common condition. According to incomplete statistics, more than 80 million people in China suffer from depression out of a population of nearly 1.4 billion (dated to 2016). Most people with depression have suicidal tendencies, so this condition is very detrimental.

Excessive emotions will lead to abnormal functions of the liver. According to 'Fundamental Questions: Significant Discussions on Phenomena Corresponding to *Yin* and *Yang*,' 'anger impairs the liver.' It can disrupt the liver's mobilization of *qi* and blood and cause abnormal functions of coursing and discharge. Then what do you do to avoid the harm of excessive emotions to the liver?

As was mentioned in a previous chapter, you can take appropriate ways to vent your emotions. For example, if you often nag your friends and family, you can divert your emotions by doing physical exercise or go to a therapist for counseling to vent. These are the ways you can choose to maintain healthy emotions and to avoid impairing the liver. If someone around you often loses temper, you could sympathize with them because they may have been stressed at work or had been staying up late recently. In this case, chatting with them would be a good way to help them vent emotions and protect the liver.

Q6. How does the liver regulate spiritual activities?

The liver can also regulate one's spiritual activities. Here, I'd like to take sleep as an example. Why is it that some people can remember a little bit of their dreams while others cannot? Why do some people talk or walk in their sleep? These are all related to what the liver does. In essence, sleep is dominated by the heart where spirit is stored. The heart spirit regulates sleep by controlling the ethereal and corporeal souls. Stored in the liver, the ethereal soul is a higher-level consciousness which can dominate the corporeal soul. The corporeal soul by contrast is stored in the lung and refers to intuitive perception. For example, when someone touches you, you can feel it. This reflects the function of the corporeal soul.

As is stated in 'Miraculous Pivot: Basic State of Spirit,' 'what comes and goes following the spirit is called ethereal soul.' When one falls asleep, the heart spirit is calm, and it has less control over the ethereal soul. Therefore, some of the ethereal soul will act independently and make the corporeal soul produce dreams. An overactive ethereal soul will receive more intense responses from the corporeal soul, such as sleepwalking, talking in the sleep. These spiritual activities come from consciousness, so the heart spirit cannot feel them.

According to this, how does TCM treat diseases with dreaminess, sleepwalking and sleeptalking? TCM doctors often use such settling tranquilizers as Raw

Dragon Bone (*shēng lóng gǔ* 生龙骨), Raw Oyster Shell (*shēng mǔ lì* 生牡蛎), and Magnetite (*cí shí* 磁石) to tranquilize the heart spirit and constrain the ethereal soul. In this way, the ethereal soul will be restrained from the dominant corporeal soul and diseases will be cured. Thus, both the liver dominating the ethereal soul and the ethereal soul dominating the corporeal soul can be the manifestations of the liver function.

Q7. How does the liver regulate digestive function?

Why do people lose their appetite when they are busy or angry? It is due to what the liver does to the spleen and stomach. According to the five-element theory, the liver is associated with wood and the spleen is associated with earth. Whether people have appetite depends on the spleen, the digestive organ. Under normal circumstances, wood restricts earth, and the regulation of *qi* by the liver can promote the digestive function of the spleen. If the liver is depressed and *qi* does not flow freely, the digestive function of the spleen will also be disturbed, resulting in loss of appetite, bloating, and other discomforts.

As is known to all, if some grass and trees grow on the land, the soil will feel soft; if there are no grass or trees, the soil will feel firm. This is called 'earth (*qi*) is loose; wood *qi* flows freely' in 'Fundamental Questions: Significant Discussions on the Administration of Five Motions' (*Sù Wèn Wǔ Cháng Zhèng Dà Lùn* 素问•五常政大论). In this sentence, 'wood *qi* flows freely' provides a premise for 'earth (*qi*) is loose.' If wood (liver) *qi* does not flow freely, earth (*qi*) will not be loose, and the spleen and stomach will have difficulty in digesting. There is another situation: if one's liver *qi* flows too freely, one will get angry and then have diarrhea. This is because liver *qi* which flows too freely may impair the spleen and stomach and accelerate gastrointestinal peristalsis. After people go to the toilet, their stomachache will be relieved.

For indigestion caused by liver depression, TCM physicians treat it by soothing the liver and strengthening the spleen. I once had a patient in his 50s who was always quiet and sulking. His most apparent symptom was a stomachache and an inability to digest hard food. The rice needed to be steamed for more than two hours before he ate it. Once, his prospective daughter-in-law came to their house and helped with cooking. The rice was not steamed for long enough because she didn't know his eating habits. He then came to see the doctor due to the worsening pain in his stomach.

His illness was caused by liver depression and spleen deficiency, so he was given a prescription called Carefree Powder (*Xiāo Yáo Sǎn* 逍遥散). The Chinese expression *xiao yao* (逍遥) indicates that one will be carefree and unfettered after taking this medicine. In the prescription, Chinese Thorowax Root (*chái hú* 柴胡), Peppermint (*bò he* 薄荷) and Fresh Ginger (*shēng jiāng* 生姜) are used to soothe the liver and regulate *qi*. White Peony Root (*bái sháo* 白芍) is used in combination with Chinese Angelica to constrain and emolliate the liver and make liver *qi* flow more freely. Poria Cocos (*fú líng* 茯苓), White Atractylodes Rhizome (*bái zhú* 白术), and Liquorice Root are used to strengthen the spleen and stomach. The entire formula is designed to soothe the liver so that the spleen and stomach can function normally, making the patient feel relieved.

Q8. How does the liver regulate reproductive function?

The liver's mobilization of *qi* is also reflected in its regulation of reproductive function. If something goes wrong with reproduction, most people would think it is caused by kidney deficiency and then try to tonify the kidney. In fact, reproductive function is also closely related to the liver. 'Miraculous Pivot: Meridians' (*Líng Shū Jīng Mài* 灵枢·经脉) states that the Liver Meridian of Foot Reverting *Yin* 'enters the pubic hair region, curves around the external genitalia, and goes up to the lower abdomen.' It shows the close relationship between the reproductive organs and the liver meridian. According to Zhu Danxi, a physician of the Yuan dynasty, 'the liver governs coursing and discharge.' It indicates that the excretion of a man's kidney essence is dominated by the liver, which also proves the close relationship between the liver and reproduction.

I had a patient in his 30s who had to take aphrodisiacs every time he had sex with his wife. Through inspection, I found that he had acne on his face, sores in his mouth, and a red tongue with yellow greasy coating. Through inquiry, I learnt that he and his wife had been married for three years and wanted to have a child. He drank a lot. His mouth was always dry with a bitter taste. He also complained that he had a damp scrotum.

He was diagnosed as dampness-heat in liver meridian, so I treated him by using the method of dispelling the dampness-heat. Here, I would like to give a piece of advice to those young men who have symptoms of impotence and premature ejaculation. If you take kidney tonics, but the effect is not significant, you should consider whether your impotence is caused by psychological or emotional factors. As mentioned above, emotional activities are regulated by the liver. When liver *qi* flows freely, psychological pressure will be relieved, and the diseases of impotence and premature ejaculation can be cured. It is unreasonable to overuse the method of tonifying the kidney.

Menstruation is also closely related to the functions of the liver. Before menstruation, some women may have distension and fullness in their breasts. They are upset, sad, and even vulnerable to tears. Their menstruation is often delayed and accompanied by severe pain. These symptoms are caused by stagnation of liver *qi*. Other women are apt to lose their temper. They often have early menstruation and suffer from metrorrhagia and metrostaxis. These symptoms are caused by exuberant liver fire. Therefore, it is an important method to treat irregular menstruation and dysmenorrhea from the aspect of the liver.

Chapter 7
General's Likes and Dislikes

Q1. What does it mean that the liver is on the left?

Some people despise TCM because they don't believe it is scientific. Once, a man who knew a few things about TCM asked me if TCM was wrong about the anatomical position of the liver. He pointed out that the liver is anatomically on the right side of the human body, but TCM states 'the liver is on the left.' Therefore, he questioned the scientific nature and clinical value of TCM theory. *Huangdi's Inner Canon of Medicine* contains a lot of anatomical information, among which the anatomical position of the liver is mentioned in the chapters of *Miraculous Pivot* such as 'The Relationship between Rivers and Channels,' 'The Viscera as the Foundation of Human Beings,' and 'Bravery.' The *Canon* does say that the liver is on the left and this view has evolved into the mainstream understanding of the liver in TCM. According to 'Fundamental Questions: Contraindication of Needling Therapy' (*Sù Wèn Cì Jìn Lùn* 素问•刺禁论), 'the liver is on the left; the lung is stored on the right; the heart commands in the exterior; the kidney governs the interior.'

The ancient Chinese locate the direction according to the following. They stand facing south because there is the sun in the south. In this way, the left is east, and the right is west. Seeing the sun rise in the east and set in the west, they think that all ascending *qi* is from the left and descending *qi* is from the right. 'Fundamental Questions: Significant Discussions on Phenomena Corresponding to *Yin* and *Yang*' states: 'The left and the right are the routes of *yang* and *yin*.' That is, *yang qi* ascends from the left while *yin qi* descends from the right. Therefore, the saying that 'the liver is on the left' doesn't mean that the liver is anatomically on the left, but that liver *qi* ascends from the left because the liver governs ascending and dispersion. Similarly, the saying that 'the lung is stored on the right' indicates that lung *qi* descends from the right because the lung governs purification and descending.

Q2. Why can liver *qi* ascend?

When asked what the most powerful thing is in the world, some say elephants, some say lions, and some say King Kong. An experiment gives the answer to this question. The human skull is remarkably intact. The edges of the bones are serrated so that the bones firmly interlock with each other, and it is hard to break it open with mechanical force. After many attempts that anatomists and physiologists made have failed, someone then suggested putting seeds in the skull, keeping them at the suitable temperature and humidity and waiting for them to germinate. Finally, the seeds germinated, and the skull was gradually opened, leaving the serrations intact. Therefore, it can be concluded that seeds are the most powerful things in the world.

In everyday life, it is not rare for you to find that the grass grows among the rubble and the trees grow on the cliffs. Zheng Banqiao (郑板桥) of the Qing dynasty (1616–1911) wrote a poem to praise bamboo: 'Upright stands the bamboo amid green mountains steep. Its toothlike root in broken rock is planted deep. It is strong and firm though struck and beaten without rest. Careless of the wind from north or south, east, or west.'[1] The poem shows the strength of bamboo and praises it for its tenacious survival in harsh conditions. In fact, the characteristics of wood in the five-element theory are summarized in analogy to those of seeds and plants. In

---

[1] The poem is titled 'Bamboo in the Rock' (*Zhú Shí* 竹石) and the English version translated by Xu Yuanchong (许洲冲 the first Chinese winner of 'Aurora Borealis' Prize) is quoted here.

the 'Great Principles' of *The Book of History*[①] (*Shàng Shū* 尚书) states: 'Wood is characterized by bending and straightening.' The germination of a seed is a process from bending to straightening, which shows the great strength of the seed. In TCM, the liver pertains to wood and is in the lower energizer. Compared to a seed, the liver also has some strength and power, pushing liver *qi* to move upward and outward. In other words, the liver mobilizes *qi* and blood and regulates *qi* circulation. Besides, the liver is the army general. Its strength can be interpreted through its similarity to the power of an army general. Hence, according to TCM, liver *qi* can ascend because it has some strength and power.

Q3. What is the liver's 'personality'?

To answer this question, let us review the theory of visceral manifestations. As you may know, the understanding of the *zang-fu* organs in TCM is not entirely based on anatomy. Visceral manifestations or *zang xiang* frame a viewpoint of TCM to understand the *zang-fu* organs. According to Zhang Jiebin, a medical scholar of the Ming dynasty, *zang* refers to the *zang-fu* organs stored in the human body while *xiang* refers to the exterior manifestations of the *zang-fu* organs. The latter can also be interpreted as the features of the *zang-fu* organs. In other words, TCM understands the *zang-fu* organs by observing their manifestations in the exterior. Thus, it can be seen that the *zang-fu* organs in TCM tend to be understood at their functional level; they don't exactly refer to the anatomical entities.

As mentioned previously, the liver governs ascending and dispersion. Its *qi* moves upward and outward and is of great strength. The liver prefers free activity and detests depression. On one hand, *qi* and blood flow freely. If *qi* and blood stagnate, the liver will be diseased. For example, *qi* and blood stasis may cause severe abdominal pain, breast distension, and emotional instability during a woman's period. In this case, it should be treated by the method of soothing the liver to enable

---

① *The Book of History*: a collection of rhetorical prose attributed to figures of ancient China and served as the foundation of Chinese political philosophy for over 2,000 years. Compiled about 3,000 years ago in the Warring States Period, it is one of the Five Classics of ancient Chinese literature.

the free flow of *qi*. On the other hand, emotions should be smooth and free from depression.

'Every month there are always a few special days.' This is a line delivered in an advertisement to refer to women's menstrual cycle. Once, a man uttered this line with a sigh, which made his colleagues roar with laughter. It reflected the man's depressed mood. Such a case calls for the therapy of regulating the mood and relieving the pressure.

'Fundamental Questions: *Qi* in the *Zang*-organs Following the Rules of Seasonal Changes' states: 'Liver *qi* needs to be dissipated. A liver disorder requires immediate consumption of pungent flavor to dissipate its *qi*. Use pungent flavors to tonify liver *qi* and sour flavors to purge it.' This sentence really puzzles many people. Tonics such as Milkvetch Root and Ginseng (*rén shēn* 人参) are often used to replenish *qi* and blood. Why does it say to tonify the liver with pungent flavor? Furthermore, sour medicinals often act as astringents. Why does it say to purge the liver with sour flavor? The truth is that liver *qi* longs for dispersion and smooth flow, and the pungent flavor induces dispersion, which agrees with the liver's personality. The sourness induces contraction and goes against the liver's character of dispersion. Hence the saying: the pungent tonifies the liver and the sour purges the liver. Stagnation of liver *qi* indicates its insufficiency or the liver's dysfunction in governing the free flow of *qi*; therefore, it should be treated by tonifying liver *qi* to restore its free flow. Pungent medicinals such as Fresh Ginger, Peppermint, and Turmeric Root Tuber (*yù jīn* 郁金) can be used to assist dispersion. In the case of excess liver fire or hyperactivity of liver *qi* characterized by anger, irritability, dry tongue, and a bitter taste in the mouth, sour medicinals can be used to astringe the liver and purge fire.

In a nutshell, the personality of the liver can be described as its preference for free activity and its dislike of depression.

Q4. What in nature corresponds to the liver?

The liver pertains to wood (element) and corresponds to east (direction) and spring (season). As the Chinese proverb goes, 'Spring is like a child that changes his emotions several times a day.' It indicates that the weather in spring is unpredictable. It may be cold in the morning and evening, but hot at noon. The temperature may rise tomorrow but fall the day after. The capricious weather makes it difficult for people to decide what to wear in springtime. Sometimes they wear coats and sometimes they wear short-sleeved shirts. Additionally, spring is also a season characterized by strong wind. Since the liver is related to spring, the liver is also believed to be closely related to wind.

Q5. What are the two characteristics of wind?

In TCM, the liver is closely related to wind. There are two main characteristics of wind: 1) wind tends to move and have frequent changes; 2) wind tends to cause vibration.

First, as is stated in 'Fundamental Questions: Wind' (*Sù Wèn Fēng Lùn* 素问·风论), 'wind tends to move and have frequent changes.' Wind comes and goes suddenly and irregularly. Sometimes it is strong whereas sometimes it is weak. Analogically, a disease with rapid development and an unfixed location is caused by a wind pathogen. A couple of diseases can be attributed to wind, for example, rubella, asthma, hives, and allergic rhinitis.

For some people, after having had a cold for two weeks and having almost recovered, one problem remains, that is, an itchy throat. They'll cough the moment their throats feel itchy, which is spontaneous and uncontrollable. The coughing stops when the itching stops. I once experienced a sudden fit of itching in my throat during in-class lecturing and couldn't manage to speak until I had a severe cough attack. I then resumed talking and had no itch or cough at all. These symptoms are manifested as sudden attack and sudden stoppage. Some people may suggest taking boiled pear with rock sugar or Dwarf Lilyturf Root (*mài dōng* 麦冬) to relieve the itchy throat and cough. But the symptoms won't be relieved by using those foods and medicinals for nourishing *yin*. Rather, this kind of sudden itchy throat and cough can be eased by medicinals for dispelling wind.

As you may know, when one is allergic, one may have itchy skin. Upon scratching, there may appear to be rashes, raised bumps or red patches on the skin.

Some of them are red, some are white, and some are pale. They will disappear after a period of time if you leave them unattended, which relates to the 'sudden-attack-and-sudden-stoppage' signs and symptoms. This skin condition is also caused by a wind pathogen and is called wind rash in TCM or rubella as it may be known to you.

Asthma can be a tricky disease and hard to treat. Asthma patients suffer a lot, and some of them even die from dyspnea caused by asthma. When there isn't an asthma attack, the patient behaves just like a normal person. Once the attack occurs, it can be difficult to control. It is also a condition characterized by sudden attack and sudden stoppage. As you may know, the lung governs *qi* and controls breathing; asthma is closely related to the lung. However, treating asthma only from the aspect of the lung is sometimes not effective.

Wu Weiping (武维屏), a professor at Dongzhimen Hospital (the First Affiliated Hospital of Beijing University of Chinese Medicine) in Beijing, believes that the sudden attack and sudden stoppage of asthma are like the characteristics of wind, so in addition to treating the lung, she tried the method of pacifying the liver and extinguishing wind. That is, she treated the liver and the lung simultaneously, which was proved to be effective. Therefore, based on inheriting the tradition, innovation is sometimes required for better results.

I had a patient in his 50s who had a disease I hadn't encountered before. He felt a rush of *qi* running through his body, sometimes to his shoulders, sometimes to his arms, sometimes to his legs, and sometimes to the acupoint *bai hui* (百会 GV 20) at the top of his head. The body part, to which the *qi* rushed, would be painful. What's more, if it was pinched or struck, the patient would have a long and loud hiccup. Every spring, he would ask others to hit him with a stick to induce hiccups and he wouldn't feel better until the hiccups stopped and the *qi* was gone. The location of the disease is not fixed, so this is what we call wind disease in TCM.

Clinically, patients with changeable emotions are also very common. I once saw a patient with manic-depressive psychosis. During the manic episode, he appeared quick-minded and had a good memory. At that time, he was preparing for the postgraduate school entrance examination. He was finally admitted to Peking University as a graduate student with excellent grades. However, after entering the school, he became depressed and showed no interest in study. He failed in many exams and finally had to drop out. The manic episode gave way to the depressive episode. The changes between mania and depression are unpredictable, so this disease also reflects the characteristics of wind, that is, sudden attack and sudden stoppage.

To sum up, wind is characterized by unpredictable movement and frequent change. It may cause some diseases with unfixed location or featured by sudden occurrence and sudden disappearance. This is the first characteristic of wind.

Second, wind tends to cause vibration. Wind scale is described in a Chinese primary textbook as follows: 'When its force is 0, smoke rises vertically; when its force is 1, smoke drifts following the wind direction; when its force is 2, wind gently touches the face; when its force is 3, leaves constantly move and flags are extended; when its force is 4, loose paper is lifted and small tree branches move; when its force is 5, small trees in leaf begin to sway; when its force is 6, umbrellas are lifted and resistance is felt when one walks against wind.' When wind blows, things such as tress, branches, and flags sway uncontrollably. As the saying goes, 'the trees desire stillness but the wind will not cease.' The constant movement due to the stirring of wind can be extended to the human body.

In TCM, wind diseases are manifested in the shaking or trembling of any body part that should remain still, or in the stiffness of any body parts that are supposed to be flexible. According to 'Fundamental Questions: Significant Discussions on the Most Important and Abstruse Theory,' 'all wind diseases characterized by shaking and dizziness are associated with the liver (*zhū fēng diào xuàn, jiē shǔ yú gān* 诸风掉眩, 皆属于肝).' Here, *diao* (掉) refers to the shaking of body parts, and *xuan* (眩) or *yun* (晕) refers to dizziness. Zhang Jiebin of the Ming dynasty explains '*yūn*' (晕 dizziness) as '*yùn*' (运 movement), which shows its similarity to the characteristic of wind. In the same text, there is another sentence: 'All syndromes characterized by sudden stiffness are associated with wind (*zhū bào jiāng zhí, jiē shǔ yú fēng* 诸暴强直, 皆属于风).' Here, *bao* (暴) means 'sudden' and *jiang zhi* (强直) indicates the stiffness of body parts such as tendons and vessels that are expected to be soft and flexible.

There is a disease called cerebral apoplexy or stroke in Western medicine. It refers to the cerebrovascular abnormalities caused by stenosis, blockage, bleeding, or rupture of blood vessels in the brain. Cerebral apoplexy can be ischemic or hemorrhagic, which is very harmful to human beings. According to incomplete statistics, there are about two million new cases of this disease in China every year. A variety of sequelae often occur after the acute stage, which does great harm to human health. Clinically, apoplexy is mainly manifested by mental disorder, movement disorder, sensory and perceptual disorder as well as language disorder. Patients with cerebral apoplexy often suddenly fall to the ground and become unconscious. Although they regain consciousness after treatment, they don't speak coherently. Some patients may suffer from hemiplegia. Their legs and feet become inflexible and cannot be raised normally. Other patients may have numb extremities. When a needle is inserted, they have little or no feeling at all. TCM believes that this disorder is caused by a wind pathogen, hence it is called wind stroke and is treated by pacifying the liver and extinguishing wind. In addition, activating blood and resolving stasis should also be used to treat the disease, because numbness of hands and feet is caused by *qi* and blood stagnation.

In clinical practice, there is another kind of wind disease called chorea minor, which usually occurs in girls aged 5–15. These patients often wink and stick their tongues out to make funny faces. Their arms are often stretched out and folded back alternately, as if they are dancing. Additionally, cerebellar ataxia makes their limbs uncoordinated and their steps clumsy. The disease, as TCM believes, is caused by the internal stirring of liver wind.

Parkinson's disease is yet another example. Muhammad Ali, one of the world's greatest boxers, had this kind of disease. Many of his symptoms are described in his daughter's book *I'll Hold Your Hand So You Won't Fall*. The characteristic symptoms are that his hands kept shaking and his steps were fast and flustered. Parkinson's disease is also caused by the internal stirring of liver wind. TCM treats it by pacifying the liver and extinguishing wind.

Some wind symptoms cannot be observed through inspection. They are simply the patient's own feelings and need to be identified through inquiry. As was mentioned above, 'Fundamental Questions: Significant Discussions on the Most Important and Abstruse Theory' states that 'all wind diseases characterized by shaking and dizziness are associated with the liver.' The patients report that they feel their heads spinning and they are sick and vomit and cannot get out of bed. While Western medicine holds that this is a disease of the inner ear, TCM ascribes it to liver wind, proposing that it should be treated from the aspect of the liver.

In fact, some cases are caused by external wind, so the method of dispelling wind should be used; some cases are caused by internal wind, so the method of pacifying the liver and extinguishing wind should be used. The two treatment methods are different. It is advised that you should visit the doctors for medical consultation when you do not feel well.

Q6. How do you nourish the liver in spring?

The liver pertains to wood. It governs ascending and dispersion and is related to the season of spring. In spring, the grass starts to turn green, the leaves start to grow, and the flowers start to blossom. 'The natural world is resuscitating, and all things are flourishing,' reads the text—'Fundamental Questions: Significant Discussions on Regulating the Spirit in Accordance with the *Qi* of the Four Seasons.' Therefore, TCM believes that *yang qi* starts to grow and tends to flourish in spring. Since spring corresponds to the liver, you should do the following to nourish the liver.

First, you should 'sleep early at night and rise early in the morning and take a walk in the courtyard with hair running free to relax the body and enliven the mind', according to 'Fundamental Questions: Significant Discussions on Regulating the Spirit in Accordance with the *Qi* of the Four Seasons.' Compared with your lifestyle in winter, you need to do more exercise in springtime to adapt to the growth of *yang qi*. The exercise should not be strenuous. Taking a walk in the courtyard can be a good choice. The ancient Chinese often have their hair tied, so it is advised that they loosen their hair to relax themselves and keep the free flow of *yang qi*. Moreover, all kinds of plans should be formulated and designed in springtime, because at that time of the year, mind begins to be activated.

Second, when dealing with things, you should adopt the principle as is described in 'Fundamental Questions: Significant Discussions on Regulating the Spirit in Accordance with the *Qi* of the Four Seasons.' During the spring season, you should 'allow things to live instead of killing, give instead of taking away, and reward instead of punishing.' No matter what happens, praise it rather than blame it. This is the way to keep a good mood and nourish the liver in spring.

Third, it is suggested that you go for an outing with your friends or family to enjoy the flourishing natural scenery in spring. In this way, you can also relax yourself and nourish your liver *qi*.

In conclusion, the above tips are generally the ways or principles for you to follow to adapt to spring *qi* and maintain your health.

Chapter 8
Causes of Fatigue

Q1. What is fatigue syndrome?

I often hear people say that they have been feeling very tired recently. A man in his 50s told me that he didn't want to do anything but sit on the couch after he came home from work. After dinner, he had to nap on the couch and then he preferred to watch soap operas. He said that he didn't need to think about anything and just had fun when he watched those programs. This is a symptom of fatigue.

Cases of fatigue are not rare. Several days ago, a woman in the outpatient department complained that she had been very tired recently and didn't feel like doing anything. Additionally, she often felt depressed and wasn't interested in anything. She also had some other symptoms including a low fever, sore throat, headache, dizziness, dysphoria, irritability, and poor appetite. Among more than 20 listed symptoms, fatigue was the most predominant one. Obviously, she suffered from what we call chronic fatigue syndrome (CFS).

CFS is now a common disorder amongst the global population. Data from CDC (Centers for Disease Control and Prevention) of the United States shows that CFS is one of the five main reasons why people go to see a doctor. Though physical examinations show no organic lesion in the patients, such symptoms are always reported as discomfort, tiredness, and fatigue. Chinese people call this state *jin pi li jin* (筋疲力尽), meaning tiredness of the sinews and exhaustion of strength.

Q2. What is the relationship between the sinews and the liver?

Some Chinese expressions contain the word 'sinew' for the description of a person with great stamina, like *jin gu hao* (筋骨好 , literally bones and sinews being good) and *jin gu qiang jin* (筋骨强劲 , literally bones and sinews being strong). According to 'Fundamental Questions: Elucidation of Five *Qi*' (*Sù Wèn Xuān Míng Wǔ Qì Piān* 素问•宣明五气篇), 'the liver governs the sinews.' *Explanation of Scripts and Elucidation of Characters* states that the sinew is the strength of the flesh. The character 筋 (*jīn*) contains flesh and strength in the lower part and bamboo in the upper part. Bamboo is a kind of plant with abundant sinews. It is hard to break a piece of bamboo into two parts because it has many filaments, which are the sinews.

In TCM, the sinews include such tissues as fascias tendons, and ligaments.

'Fundamental Questions: Special Discussion on Meridians and Vessels' (*Sù Wèn Jīng Mài Bié Lùn* 素问•经脉别论) states that 'food and drinks enter the stomach, and the essence is then transmitted to the liver; the excessive liver *qi* flows to nourish the sinews.' In other words, after water and food we intake are digested and transformed into essence, some essence will be transported to nourish the liver. Then, the liver mobilizes these nutrients to nourish and strengthen the sinews. As was mentioned in the previous chapters, the liver is the general and the heart is the monarch governing the mind. The liver would mobilize *qi* and blood to reach the fascias that exert strength by following the heart. *Qi* and blood will flow to the legs and feet when one climbs the stairs or hills, and to the arms and hands when one lifts things.

Hence, the wellness of sinews and strength are closely related to the liver, and fatigue occurs when one's sinews get tired, and strength is exhausted.

Q3. What happens to your sinews if the liver undergoes pathological changes?

If the liver undergoes pathological changes and fails to mobilize *qi* and blood in your body, then your sinews can't help you complete tasks such as climbing hills or lifting things. You will feel tired easily.

Some people even have limb numbness. That is, they want to perform certain movements with their hands, legs, or feet, but their sinews can't receive commands and they cannot move flexibly. This state is called the inhibited flexion and extension, usually accompanied by numbness of joints.

I once treated a patient with such limb problems in the outpatient department. He was more than 50 years old and came from Northeast China. He worked in a parking lot along a narrow street in Beijing. The drivers needed to pay when they left the parking lot. Initially, there was no fee-collecting machine and the man sometimes had to ride his bike to collect a parking fee. But after sitting or standing for a while, he had a problem of stiff legs, and it was hard for him to move right away. Once, he fell as soon as he got on the bike when he was going to chase a car which was about to leave.

He had been treated many times in the Affiliated Hospital of Harbin Medical University, and the diagnosis was eosinophilic fasciitis. It is an autoimmune disease that the increase of eosinophilic cells leads to diffuse fasciitis of nerves and fascia, which is mainly manifested as impaired limb activity with numbness and pain. After various treatments by Western medicine, he was told that his disease couldn't be cured, and he had to rest at home. Helplessly, he phoned his boss and said he wouldn't return to Beijing since he had to stay at home due to his disease. The boss recommended him to come to Beijing for second opinions. Then, the man came back to Beijing with a glimmer of hope.

He came to my consultation room with others' support because he couldn't walk by himself, let alone sit or lie down. I found he had *bi*-syndrome, a case of fascia injury. It is stated in 'Fundamental Questions: *Bi*-syndrome' (*Sù Wèn Bì Lùn* 素问•痹论) that 'the mingling of pathogenic wind, cold, and dampness causes impediment or obstruction.' In other words, the three kinds of pathogens, or in TCM, the pathogenic *qi*, that is, wind, cold and dampness, invade the human body together, resulting in *bi*-syndrome combined with disordered flow of *qi* and blood in the body. *Bi*-syndrome means obstruction of *qi* and blood circulation and blockage in the meridians and collaterals. As a result, the fascias lack nourishment and are impeded by the pathogenic factors, hence leading to the occurrence of those symptoms such as rigidity, inflexibility, and pain of the limbs.

Accordingly, I treated this patient by eliminating cold and dampness, nourishing blood, and emolliating the liver. One month later, the patient could come to my consultation room on his own. After another two months, the man went back to work in the parking lot. He could also walk or ride a bike to the drivers to collect parking fees. This case may sound incredible, but the mechanism is not difficult to understand. I treated it from the aspect of the liver as the liver governs the sinews.

Some elder people may stumble due to their inflexible limbs, and their walking gait is different from what it was when they were in their youths. According to 'Fundamental Questions: Genuine *Qi* Endowed by Heaven in Remote Antiquity,' liver *qi* weakens as people get older. It says that for men 'at the age of 56, liver *qi* declines and the sinews become inflexible.' It means that when people reach a certain age of about 56 years old, liver *qi* is insufficient; hepatic blood thus fails to nourish the sinews. Then, signs and symptoms such as teetering gait, limb numbness, and difficulty moving may occur.

Q4. How do you strengthen the sinews?

Since the sinews govern movement and they are attached to your joints with connecting function, you should have more physical activities. Only with more activities can *qi* and blood reach the sinews to nourish them. Lack of physical activity can impair the circulation of *qi* and blood, and it will be difficult for *qi* and blood to reach them. If the sinews are deprived of nutrition and nourishment for a long time, the joints will not be flexible when they move. Therefore, you should work out regularly.

But remember to avoid excessive activity. You may have such an experience that after a long time you haven't tried mountain climbing, you will be exhausted with sore lower back and leg pains when you climb a mountain occasionally. The reason is that the sinews are overused, bringing on insufficiency of *qi* and blood and their failure to nourish them. According to 'Miraculous Pivot: Nine Needles' (*Líng Shū Jiǔ Zhēn Lùn* 灵枢•九针论), 'protracted walking injures tendons,' which is harmful to your body. Thus, you need to do proper exercise in a moderate manner.

In addition, you need to have enough rest. According to 'Fundamental Questions: Various Relationships of the Five *Zang*-Organs,' 'when one lies down, the blood flows into the liver.' Since it is the liver that mobilizes *qi* and blood to reach the fascias, you can't harm the liver. You have to ensure adequate rest for the repairing and regulation of *qi* and blood, and then you can proceed to do some work.

Q5. What is the relationship between the eyes and the liver?

TCM believes that the liver governs the eyes. 'Miraculous Pivot: Natural Span of Life' (*Líng Shū Tiān Nián* 灵枢•天年) states that 'when one is 50 years old, liver *qi* begins to decline... vision begins to blur.' That is, when people reach their 50s, liver *qi* weakens, which is first manifested as poor vision. In addition, 'Miraculous Pivot: Length of Meridians' states that 'liver *qi* flows to the eyes and only when the liver is in harmony can the eyes differentiate the five colors.' In other words, only when liver *qi* is vigorous and its function is active, can *qi* and blood enter your eyes and you will have good eyesight.

Dry eyes and blurred vision are two of the main signs and symptoms of fatigue. Some people cannot see things clearly, they are not willing to open their eyes, and some even suffer from watery eyes. Some of them feel as if that their eyes were salted, rough and aching, and must be washed to feel better. Some people, especially females, reported that their eyes felt astringent and only eyedrops or artificial tears could help, but the symptoms would recur after a period of time. Meanwhile, they also had a dry throat. Many people think presbyopia is caused by aging because they had good vision when they were young. There is a saying: 'When you are 48 years old or so, your vision might be blurred.' You once didn't need to wear glasses, but now you have to use them to see everything. My wife, a doctor in a large hospital, is a typical case with eye issues. She had good eyesight when she was young. But now, she has five or six pairs of reading glasses and uses them to see objects that are close. Whenever necessary, she has to search for them on her office table, in her white coat pocket, somewhere at home, or in the drawer, where there are different pairs.

Some of you are nearsighted and have to wear glasses. But now due to presbyopia, you have to take off glasses when you try to see clearly something near you. That is quite inconvenient. Along with failing eyesight, fatigue also sets in with age.

In the early days when People's Republic of China was founded, people lacked food and clothes. Meat was in short supply and most people were malnourished, so night blindness was prevalent in the early 1950s. Patients who suffered from this disease could see things in the daytime, but not at night. Some people believe this is due to vitamin A deficiency. For TCM doctors, they usually use *Yang Gan Pill* (*Yáng Gān Wán* 羊肝丸) to treat this disease, together with Chinese Angelica, Barbary Wolfberry Fruit or Goji Berry (*gǒu qǐ zǐ* 枸杞子) and White Peony Root. Composed of lamb liver and Golden Thread, *Yang Gan* Pill clears heat, and it is very effective. The rationale behind this herbal formula is that the liver governs the eyes. It makes sense to eat animals' livers to prevent eye diseases. The ancient Chinese believed that *Yang Gan* Pill could cure eye diseases and eating animals' livers could help nourish the liver and improve eyesight. But caution should be taken against overconsumption.

To prevent tiredness and fatigue and to protect the liver, you should boost nutrition. For example, when stewing chicken, you can add some Chinese Angelica, White Peony Root, Goji Berry, and Tangshen (*dǎng shēn* 党参). They can enhance nutrition. However, old and frail people with fatigue symptoms need to be cautioned against overtaking the herbs. For those who do not have these fatigue symptoms, it is better to use herbal medicine as little as possible, because every medicine has its side effects, so stop using medicines when symptoms are improved. Excessiveness is nothing but harmful.

Q6. What is the five-wheel theory in ophthalmology of TCM?

Huangdi's Inner Canon of Medicine advocates holism. It is proposed that there should be a smaller whole within a big whole. For example, the five elements include wood, fire, earth, metal, and water, and each element also consists of another five elements. This is called 'five elements storing each other' in TCM. Take the face, for instance. The face is dominated by the heart. But the face has many partitions that are particularly related to different *zang-fu* organs. Specifically, the ophryon is related to the lung (metal), the root of the nose to the heart (fire), the nose bridge to the liver (wood), the tip of the nose to the spleen (earth), and the lower part of the cheek to the kidney (water), respectively.

Patients who go to see TCM doctors are always asked to open the mouth to exhibit the tongue, which is dominated by the heart, for examination. If they have teeth marks on the edges of their tongue, the doctor may tell them it is a sign of spleen deficiency. A red tongue tip is the sign of heart problems because the tongue tip is associated with the heart. Thick coating on the root of the tongue shows kidney problems because this part is related to the kidney. In other words, the tongue can reflect the condition of the heart, but each subdivision is specifically related to one of the five elements and its corresponding *zang*-organ. The same is true with the eyes.

Let's go back to the concept that the liver governs the eyes. The eyes are related to the liver and liver *qi* flows to the eyes. If the liver is healthy, the eyes can distinguish the five colors. As is stated in 'Miraculous Pivot: Great Perplexity,' 'the essential *qi* of the five *zang*-organs and the six *fu*-organs all flow upwards into the eyes to enable the eyes to see.' That is to say, the essence, *qi*, and blood of the *zang-fu* organs all contribute to the formation of your eyes so that your eyes are capable of distinguishing different colors.

As was mentioned above, the eyes are governed by the liver; meanwhile, according to the theory of the five elements storing each other, the eyes can be subdivided into five portions, and each corresponds to one of the five elements and one of the five *zang*-organs. In particular, the upper and lower eyelids correspond to the spleen (earth), which are called the flesh wheel later in history. The white parts of the eyes correspond to the lung (metal), known as the *qi* wheel. The black parts of the eyes correspond to the liver (wood), known as the wind wheel. The inner and outer canthi correspond to the heart, known as the blood wheel. The central areas of your eyes, the pupils, correspond to the kidney, known as the water wheel. The flesh wheel, wind wheel, *qi* wheel, blood wheel, and water wheel are the well-known five wheels in ophthalmology of TCM. (See Figure 8-1)

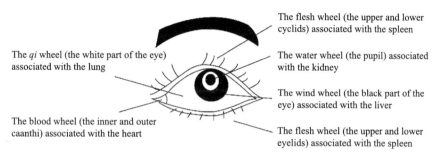

The flesh wheel (the upper and lower cyclids) associated with the spleen

The *qi* wheel (the white part of the eye) associated with the lung

The water wheel (the pupil) associated with the kidney

The wind wheel (the black part of the eye) associated with the liver

The blood wheel (the inner and outer caanthi) associated with the heart

The flesh wheel (the upper and lower eyelids) associated with the spleen

Figure 8-1   The five wheels in TCM ophthalmology

The five-wheel theory is extremely instructive for clinical practice. Here is an example. Someone gets styes. The upper eyelid is swollen and there is a small mass which is red and painful under the upper eyelid. TCM believes that there is stagnated heat in the patient's spleen and stomach because the eyelids where there is a mass are related to the spleen and stomach problems, so the treatment should be clearing the heat in the spleen and stomach. Another symptom is that some people cannot lift up their upper eyelids. Spleen *qi* is characterized by ascending and the eyelids should be able to lift. If they cannot, it means their spleen *qi* is deficient. So, in this case, in order to raise spleen *qi*, Center-tonifying *Qi*-replenishing Decoction (*Bǔ Zhōng Yì Qì Tāng* 补中益气汤) is commonly used.

Elderly people often develop cataracts as they get older. People with cataracts always feel their pupils are shielded with a thin membrane. In this case, the kidney should be tonified because the pupils are related to it.

What other eye diseases may people contract? A few years ago, people often got pinkeye in summer and their white parts of the eyes were found red. Redness of the eyeball is the manifestation of internal heat, and the white part of the eye is associated with the lung. So that means there is heat in the lung, which should be treated by medicinals to clear lung heat.

Nowadays, people spend too much time on computers and cell phones and eyestrain is caused by overuse of the eyes. Furthermore, if they keep the same posture for a long time, they may develop habitually poor posture and it may cause impairment to their eyes, liver, and other affected areas. 'Miraculous Pivot: Nine Needles' states clearly that 'protracted seeing impairs the blood.' In other words, prolonged screen time negatively affects liver blood. People should remember to investigate the distance at intervals when they are writing, using the computer or their mobile phone. They can also do eye exercises to ease eyestrain.

Q7. What is the relationship between the gallbladder and the liver?

There is a Chinese idiom *gan dan xiang zhao* (肝胆相照 , literally the liver and the gallbladder being always together), meaning utter devotion to one another. It shows that the liver and the gallbladder are intimate partners. According to *Huangdi's Inner Canon of Medicine*, the liver is the *zang*-organ while the gallbladder is the *fu*-organ, and the liver governs the gallbladder.

The gallbladder plays an important role in storing the refined juice or bile which promotes digestion. Hence, 'Miraculous Pivot: Acupoints' (*Líng Shū Běn Shū* 灵枢•本输) states that the gallbladder is 'the *fu*-organ of refined juice.' If the bile has difficulty flowing out of the liver, you will start to experience poor appetite, nausea, and vomiting.

Additionally, there is another important role of the gallbladder. 'Fundamental Questions: Secret Canon Stored in the Royal Library' states that 'the gallbladder is the justice officer, in charge of decision making.' It means that the gallbladder has an impact on one's mind when one determines whether something can or will be done or not. If gallbladder *qi* is insufficient, the decision-making function of the gallbladder will be weakened, which makes one appear indecisive. Conversely, when its function of decision making is normal, one will have courage to challenge anything whatever it is. Chinese people may say one has a small gallbladder, meaning the person is timid, or one has a big gallbladder, meaning the person is bold. Here 'gallbladder' means courage.

Justice officer is an official title, which was created in the Qin and Han dynasties, after the peasant uprising of Chen Sheng (陈胜) and Wu Guang (吴广). Justice officers are responsible for recommending talented people to the key posts of the government. Usually, they are from the noble class and are impartial. They play a key role in the country's destiny. This system is called 'recommending talents noted for their filial piety and moral records' in Chinese history.

With the development of society, this system was later abolished because of its own weaknesses. After the reign of Emperor Yang of Sui (who ruled between 604 and 618), the imperial examination system was gradually established to replace the justice officer practice. However, the statement that 'the gallbladder is the justice officer' remains. This saying shows that TCM attaches great importance to the gallbladder's function of decision making.

According to 'Fundamental Questions: Six-Plus-Six System and the Manifestations of the Viscera,' 'all eleven *zang-fu* organs depend on the gallbladder to bring their roles into full play.' It means that all *zang-fu* organs are closely associated with the gallbladder's function of decision making. Namely, all *zang-fu* organs work together when one thinks about something, but the gallbladder matters most in terms of decision making. Consequently, when somebody is indecisive and has difficulty in deciding, it is usually thought that their gallbladder's function of decision making may go wrong. In this case, the symptom is relatively mild, and physicians can alleviate it by treating the gallbladder. If the symptoms become serious, obsessive-compulsive disorder (OCD) may arise.

Patients with OCD are usually very distressed. For example, one of my friends told me that he once made an appointment with another person to do something together. When he arrived at the meeting place at the appointed time, the other man did not show up. He called up that man twice, and every time that man said that he was on his way to the appointed place. In fact, the place for them to meet was not far from that man's home. It was only about 20 minutes' walk. But my friend was kept waiting for a long time. Later, my friend asked that man what had happened. It turned out that the man had returned home twice after he left home. When he took the elevator and arrived at the ground floor, he doubted whether he had locked the door and he went back to make sure that it was locked. Then, when he reached the community gate, he doubted whether he had closed the windows and he went back again for a double check. That's why he was late for the appointment.

OCD sufferers are not uncommon. For example, one of my patients washed his hands constantly, though the skin was almost peeling. On another occasion, I had treated a female patient, a white-collar worker, who always thought that she had left something somewhere. Once I felt her pulse and gave her a prescription. Before taking the prescription to the dispensary, she picked up the wrist cushion and examined the coat hanger in my room repeatedly to see whether she had left something there. The patient acknowledged that she knew she didn't leave any personal belongings at those places, but she was just seized by a compulsion to double check it.

The obsession and compulsion bring on great distress to the patient. In fact, this is a phenomenon of compulsion and counter compulsion. Even though the patient knew what she was doing was meaningless, she felt a compulsion to reconfirm what she had done and make certain that she didn't leave anything. This is one of the characteristics of OCD.

Q8. How can obsessive-compulsive disorder (OCD) be treated?

According to TCM, OCD means insufficiency of gallbladder *qi*, namely, gallbladder deficiency. As was mentioned earlier, the liver governs the gallbladder. So, this disease can be treated by regulating the liver and the gallbladder.

A famous TCM prescription, Bupleurum and Scutellaria Gallbladder-warming Decoction (*Chái Qín Wēn Dǎn Tāng* 柴芩温胆汤), can soothe the liver and disinhibit the gallbladder, regulate *qi*, resolve phlegm, and harmonize the spleen and the stomach. The above-mentioned symptoms such as anxiety, timidity, and indecisiveness will be significantly relieved by soothing liver *qi* and gallbladder *qi* with this decoction. Meanwhile, some herbs are used to regulate the spleen and stomach, including Chinese Thorowax Root, Baical Skullcap Root, Immature Orange Fruit (*zhǐ shí* 枳实), Bamboo Shavings (*zhú rú* 竹茹), Poria Cocos, Pinellia

Tuber, and Dried Tangerine Peel (*chén pí* 陈皮). The formula works effectively to relieve indecisiveness and timidity and helps those who are easily frightened upon hearing thunder or a door close suddenly, as well as those with poor appetite and abdominal distension.

The patients who are irresolute and depressive and even have potential OCD are always found to have liver and gallbladder problems. OCD patients normally experience fatigue, vexation, and irritability before the onset of other symptoms. The conflict between compulsion and counter compulsion can cause anxiety, distress, and even physical and mental exhaustion. Some patients may feel too painful to pay any attention to work commitments. For these cases, physicians should treat them properly from the aspect of the liver and the gallbladder.

Q9. What are the causes of fatigue?

As was mentioned above, the liver is closely associated with the sinews among the five body constituents, the eyes among the five sense organs, and the gallbladder among the six *fu*-organs. So, tiredness, fatigue, blurred vision, poor appetite, repetitive thinking, indecisiveness, and anxiety are all related to the dysfunction of the liver.

That is why 'Fundamental Questions: Six-Plus-Six System and the Manifestations of the Viscera' states '*gan zhe, pi ji zhi ben*' (肝者，罢极之本), meaning the liver is the root of fatigue. Here, the Chinese character 罢 (*pí*) has the same pronunciation and meaning as 疲 (*pí*, fatigue). The character 极 (*jí*) also means tiredness and fatigue. As is stated in *Huangdi's Inner Canon of Medicine*, the root cause of fatigue is associated with liver disorder.

Q10. How do you combat fatigue?

Many people struggle with fatigue. Here are three ways for you to cope with it.

First, do proper physical exercise and get adequate rest. Try to strike a balance between work and rest. You may take a walk or play gentle sports in your free time.

Do not overstrain yourself. Have adequate rest at proper time so that the liver can have time to regulate *qi* and blood properly.

Second, alleviate mental pressure and keep a good mood. What you need to do first is to subdivide your goals into smaller tasks and to make your goals more specific. For example, you may have set yourself a 50-year goal. I am afraid such a long-term goal would bring you pressure. I advise you to turn this 50-year goal into weekly, monthly, and yearly ones and then try your best to achieve them one by one. You will feel happy when you attain these specific and short-term goals. Apart from that, do not compare with others. It is recommended that you compare your strengths with others' weaknesses if you wish to, which will allow you to have a sense of fulfillment. You can also try to find the small joys in your life.

Third, nourish the liver by enhancing nutrition. To enrich nutrition, it does not necessarily mean you eat fish and various meats. You may consider using food as a method for regulation. Many Chinese herbs can be used as food therapies. For example, you may add some Chinese Angelica, White Peony Root, Goji Berry, and Tangshen when making chicken stew. Such dishes can nourish and emolliate the liver to maintain normal function of the liver and bring vitality back to you.

Chapter 9

The Connection Between the Liver and Mood

Q1. What are the differences between men and women?

Some people say that the most prominent difference between men and women is that women experience menstruation, lactation, pregnancy, childbirth and even breastfeeding in their life, while men do not. According to *Huangdi's Inner Canon of Medicine*, the key difference between them is that women are *yin* while men are *yang* in terms of gender. *Yang* is characterized by outward, upward, bold, and rough qualities, and *yin* is inward, downward, gentle, implicit, and sensitive. Men tend to be more straightforward while women tend to be more sensitive.

Here, I would like to share a story with you to illustrate this point. There is a young couple who both have a habit of keeping a diary, from which we can see how different they are. The woman's diary reads like this. Her husband behaved weirdly that day. They made an appointment to have a meal together; however, the woman was late due to going shopping with her friends. When she finally showed up, her husband was very angry and ignored her though she apologized for being late. After the meal, she pleaded for forgiveness by saying sorry and showing love on their way home, but it didn't work. Therefore, the woman drowned herself in agony and sorrow. She cried and thought that her husband didn't love her anymore. Before going to bed, she apologized again to her husband who continued to ignore her and just focused on watching TV. When she asked her husband to go to bed, the man said that he would sleep later. She was so depressed that she thought her life would be meaningless without her husband's love and she even wanted to take her own life. By contrast, her husband's diary contained only a few words, saying 'Shit! Italy lost the game today!' The man was depressed simply because his favorite team lost in a soccer match. Unfortunately, the woman experienced big mood swings from hoping for forgiveness to depression, then to devastated crying, and finally to her loss of interest in life. This anecdote shows that men and women are quite different in personalities as they have different ways of expressing emotions and possess characteristics of their own.

Q2. What are the characteristics of women?

Women are *yin*, and blood is the basis of some physiological activities throughout their life cycle. Menstruation is their most significant characteristic. In addition, pregnancy, childbirth, and breastfeeding also depend heavily on the supply of blood. *Huangdi's Inner Canon of Medicine* states that women in general have excessive *qi* and insufficient blood. Why is this so? 'Frequent consumption of blood' is the reason. Women experience loss of blood in many circumstances such as menstruation, pregnancy, labor, and even breastfeeding. The frequent loss of blood throughout her life is precisely a particularly distinguished feature of women. It might explain why women do not grow beard like men. In a word, TCM believes that compared with men, women tend to be in a state of blood insufficiency and their *qi* is relatively excessive.

As you may know, *qi* in excess will turn into fire, so women are more likely to experience mood swings and irritability and tend to nag more than men. Furthermore, due to blood consumption and loss from time to time, women are especially prone to blood deficiency and blood stasis, which can cause dysmenorrhea, irregular menstruation, and breast hyperplasia. Chloasma may develop in those who have given birth to children or later in life. The above-mentioned symptoms and changeable moods are related to women's particular characteristics, that is, relative insufficiency of blood and excess of *qi*, closely associated with the function of the liver as the liver is believed to be the sea of blood. The liver is like an army general that mobilizes *qi* and blood in the human body and regulates *qi* and blood as well as one's mood since it governs the free flow of *qi*. Hence, the liver is believed in TCM to be most closely linked to a woman's health.

Q3. What is the relationship between mood and the liver?

I once treated a 40-year-old female patient who complained of headache, dizziness, body aches, and insomnia, but her emotional issue was the main problem. She was irritable, short-tempered, and nagging, looking unkindly on almost everything. What she used to tolerate could now easily irritate her. Upon hearing those complaints, I asked her some questions about her menstruation. She reported that she had irregular periods, sometimes earlier than expected and sometimes later. Additionally, the quantity and color of her menses were not the same as before. Those are the symptoms of menopause.

Climacterium, written as 更年期 (*gēng nián qī*) in Chinese, is a particular phase in a female's life cycle. The Chinese character 更 (*gēng*) means replacing or substituting, and 年 (*nián*) means age bracket. When do females have their first menstruation? According to 'Fundamental Questions: Genuine *Qi* Endowed by Heaven in Remote Antiquity,' for a female 'at the age of 14, *tian gui* (天癸) matures; conception vessel is passable; thoroughfare vessel is vigorous; period occurs in due time. Hence, she can conceive a baby.' *Tian gui*, a TCM term, refers to the substance that promotes the development of reproductive system or the sex-stimulating substance. It is governed by the kidney. After *tian gui* is matured, conception vessel and thoroughfare vessel become vigorous, and a girl thus starts to have menstruation. Menstruation is called 月事 (*yuè shì*) in Chinese, which literally translates as monthly event or matter. Its occurrence signifies that a girl can conceive a baby. In other words, her body reaches reproductive maturity.

Then, after several decades, women experience the transition from physical maturity to degeneration. 'Fundamental Questions: Genuine *Qi* Endowed by Heaven in Remote Antiquity' states that 'at the age of 49, conception vessel becomes deficient; thoroughfare vessel weakens and diminishes; *tian gui* is exhausted and menstruation ceases. Hence, she becomes physically feeble and is no longer able to conceive a baby.' When women are 49 years old, *tian gui*, the substance that can promote the growth, development, and reproduction of the human body, is in decline, resulting in the lack of *qi* and blood in the conception vessel and the thoroughfare vessel. The significant signs are menopause and the loss of fertility. Therefore, climacterium refers to the time period around menopause, during which a female's fertility goes from maturity to degeneration.

Symptoms such as hot flushes, sweating, dizziness, headaches, and insomnia usually occur during one's menopausal transition. Most evident of all are emotional changes, including irritability, restlessness, and a tendency to lose one's temper and feel frustrated.

Climacterium is something that all women have to experience. Females should face the transition calmly and treat it as a natural part of their lives. Of course, they should go to see doctors when they feel unwell. *Huangdi's Inner Canon of Medicine* states that the kidney is mainly responsible for reproduction, and menopause is related to the exhaustion of *tian gui* which heavily depends on kidney *qi*. However, the liver also plays an important role. It is especially true when it comes to the formation of menstruation. Since the blood in the conception vessel and the thoroughfare vessel flows downward into the uterus to form menses, attention should also be paid to liver regulation.

What's more important is that women tend to be emotionally unstable, tend to be irritated due to their relative excess of *qi*, and tend to experience mood swings during menopausal transition—all of these are related to the liver. *Huangdi's Inner Canon of Medicine* classifies human emotions into seven kinds: joy, anger, anxiety, overthinking, sorrow, fear, and fright, all of which are generally governed by the heart (the organ like a monarch) and specifically managed by the liver (the organ similar to an army general). Therefore, one important function of the liver is regulating emotions. According to this theory, when there are signs and symptoms of emotional changes, physicians should consider the treatment from the liver aspect. The liver pertains to wood among the five elements. Wood is associated with wind, which is capricious, uncertain, and unpredictable. So, by analogy, it is common that someone tends to be irritable and capricious in their emotions. For instance, one may suddenly cheer up during a quarrel, or suddenly get angry during a happy conversation. This kind of phenomenon is associated with wind in nature according to TCM, and wind pertains to the liver. Thus, TCM states that the liver is the basis for females. In simple words, the liver is most closely linked to a woman's health.

Q4. What is the relationship between menstruation and the liver?

Menstruation is a gender characteristic of women. It has a close relationship with pregnancy or gestation. Menstruation and its condition have a close relationship with reproduction.

When kidney *qi* becomes abundant at the age of 14 in a female, *tian gui*, the substance which promotes the maturity of reproductive function, also becomes mature, leading to the development of reproductive system and the abundance of blood in the thoroughfare vessel and the conception vessel. The liver regulates and controls the blood in the two vessels. Therefore, the liver has a close relationship with menstruation as well as the kidney.

When there are menstrual disorders, treatment should focus on the aspect of the liver. The reasons are as follows:

First, the basis for the formation of menses comes from the liver. The blood in the thoroughfare vessel and the conception vessel flows downwards into the uterus and menstruation occurs. But how does the blood in the thoroughfare vessel and the conception vessel come into being? It is liver blood, for the liver is the sea of blood and it stores blood.

Second, the condition of menstruation is closely linked to the function of the liver. The liver is an organ like an army general that regulates the circulation of *qi* and blood. When the period is coming, it helps the blood in the thoroughfare vessel and the conception vessel flow to the uterus. Therefore, the liver is closely related to menstrual condition.

Third, the liver regulates emotions. Mood has a significant impact on the circulation of *qi* and blood. Therefore, patients with menstrual irregularities should be treated by soothing the liver.

Q5. How can menstrual irregularities be treated?

Menstruation is expected to arrive regularly. Li Shizhen, a great TCM doctor of the Ming dynasty, made a clear statement concerning the regularity of menstruation. He suggested that menstruation cycle corresponds to *tai yin* (太阴 , referring to the moon) from heaven and to tide on earth. In a month, the moon waxes and wanes; the tide ebbs and flows. Correspondingly, menstruation occurs once a month. Hence, menstruation is called *yue jing* (月经 , literally monthly regularity) in Chinese. The Chinese character 经 (*jīng*) means regularity. It is also called *yue xin* (月信 , literally monthly message) and *yue shui* (月水 , literally monthly water) in TCM. These Chinese expressions indicate that menstruation is expected to occur on time and usually once a month. A teenage girl might miss it since that likely indicates the immaturity of the reproductive system. Meanwhile, a teenage girl may also be afraid of the arrival of a period since it may cause many problems such as dysmenorrhea, delayed menstruation, advanced menstruation, profuse menstruation, scant menstruation, and distending fullness in the breasts, chest, and hypochondria before menstruation. All these problems are generally categorized as menstrual irregularities.

Huangdi's Inner Canon of Medicine states that menstrual irregularities should be treated from the aspect of the liver. 'Fundamental Questions: Abdominal Diseases' (*Sù Wèn Fù Zhōng Lùn* 素问•腹中论) reads: 'The disease is named blood exhaustion. It is acquired in one's younger years due to massive loss of blood. Or, when one has sex in a state of drunkenness, one's *qi* is exhausted, and the liver is harmed. Hence, her menses are scant or even cease.' Here it is stated that amenorrhea and menstrual irregularities are mainly caused by liver impairment. A prescription is provided to treat it, that is, Cuttlefish Bone and Indian Madder Root Pill (*Wū*

Zéi Gǔ Lǔ Rú Wán 乌贼骨蘆茹丸). It is used to tonify the kidney, promote blood circulation, and dredge meridians. As the formula name suggests, Cuttlefish Bone (*wū zéi gǔ* 乌贼骨 / *hǎi piāo xiāo* 海螵蛸) and Indian Madder Root (*lǔ rú* 蘆茹 / *qiàn cǎo* 茜草) are the chief ingredients. The former is salty in flavor and warm in property, so it can promote menstruation and tonify blood, and thus is used for blood exhaustion and amenorrhea. The latter, bitter in flavor and cold in property, can promote blood circulation, regulate *qi*, and unblock the meridian. This prescription also contains sparrow's eggs, used to tonify the essence, reinforce essential *qi*, and nourish blood. Besides, one is recommended to take the pills with abalone soup, which is warm in property and particularly acts on the liver meridian to nourish blood.

Huangdi's Inner Canon of Medicine contains only 13 prescriptions and one of them is specially formulated to treat menstrual irregularities from the aspect of the liver, which shows the important role that the liver plays in a woman's health.

TCM believes that the liver should be emphasized in the treatment for menstrual irregularities. In clinical practice, menstrual irregularities can be treated not only with Cuttlefish Bone and Indian Madder Root Pill, but with medicinals that can regulate the liver, soothe the liver, nourish blood, and emolliate the liver.

No offense, but I would like to remind women of something concerning their clothing. Nowadays, a type of jeans, called tight pants, is popular. It is wrapped tightly on legs. However, women should not wear tight jeans during their period, as the circulations of *qi* and blood are turbulent during those days. Wearing tight jeans may worsen the condition.

I would also like to give some suggestions to men since the period is something unique to women and men cannot experience what women are suffering. Some women tend to be irritable during their menstruation. Some may experience menstrual cramps or extremely painful periods. In those circumstances, men should try to understand them and be tolerant enough to avoid having a quarrel with them.

Q6. What are the dos and don'ts during your menstrual period?

The following are the three basic things you should do to help you maintain health and prevent menstrual disorders.

First, maintain emotional stability and try to keep a mellow mood. Stay away from negative stimuli.

Second, avoid overstraining. Do not do intense physical activities.

Third, do not expose yourself to pathogenic factors. Avoid going out in adverse weather during your menstrual period. If it is very cold, wet, or rainy, you'd better stay indoors.

Here is an example to illustrate the importance of avoiding cold during one's period. I once treated a 30-year-old patient from Zhejiang province. On a winter day she had a quarrel with her husband during her period. She was so angry that she went out to dig up lotus roots in the field. The water was very cold at that time of the year. Everyone would feel bitterly cold even in leather clothes if they went to the field and dug up lotus roots. From then on, she always felt intermittently cold and hot, had poor appetite, abdominal distention, and fullness, and was easily vexed and angry. It was due to the unsmooth flow of liver *qi* and insufficiency of liver blood during the period, and then when cold and dampness invaded her body, the condition worsened, leading to *qi* stagnation and blood stasis. Finally, menstrual irregularities occurred. It was not easy to cure her because dampness, as you may know, is sticky and greasy in property and it is difficult to be removed. Therefore, medicines should be prescribed on one hand to sooth the liver, regulate *qi*, and nourish blood, and on the other hand, to remove cold and dampness. In any case, women should avoid contracting pathogenic factors during the period.

Q7. What are the causes of infertility?

Many factors can contribute to infertility. The prime cause may be kidney problems. In this chapter, I have repeatedly cited the quote in *Huangdi's Inner Canon of Medicine*, which indicates what a 14-year-old girl would experience in terms of physiological activities. As is said in 'Fundamental Questions: Genuine *Qi* Endowed by Heaven in Remote Antiquity,' for a female 'at the age of 14, *tian gui* matures; conception vessel is passable; thoroughfare vessel is vigorous; period occurs in due time. Hence, she can conceive a child.' *Tian gui*, the substance that promotes the development of reproductive system, will mature, and be governed by the kidney. Periods come regularly on time, so women have the possibility to get pregnant and bear children. The role of the liver should be taken into consideration because gestation has a close relationship with the liver. The liver can control the *qi* and blood in the thoroughfare vessel and the conception vessel to flow downwards into the uterus and nourish the fetus. If the female suffers from depression and other emotional problems, it will greatly affect gestation. In *Fu Qingzhu's Obstetrics and Gynecology*[①] (*Fù Qīng Zhǔ Nǚ Kē* 傅青主女科), it is recorded that 'patients with depression are unable to carry a fetus due to constraint of liver *qi*.' In other words, depression will cause liver dysfunction in smoothing and discharging. Since the liver fails to function well, the door to the uterus may be closed so that *qi* and blood cannot enter the uterus to nourish the fetus. Thus, to the newlyweds and those who plan to have children, it is suggested that they keep a good mood and do not put too much pressure on themselves. That is, too much stress affects pregnancy.

Here is a story about a scientist couple in a movie called 'The Law of Attraction' to illustrate the impact of pressure or stress on pregnancy. The couple used mathematical formula to calculate the exact time when the wife might get pregnant, and they would have to wait for that time to have sex. Apart from this, they tracked her basal body temperature, made recipes for boosting fertility and even prepared a sex-position power bed. It sounds somewhat crazy and absurd, doesn't it? Sadly, the wife could not get pregnant. At the end of the film, the couple gave up doing those things including making the plan for a pregnancy via medical assistance. They made love naturally. Eventually, the wife got pregnant. This story shows that stress will reduce the chances of pregnancy.

The following is a real-life case of pressure causing infertility. One day a patient

---

① *Fu Qingzhu's Obstetrics and Gynecology*: a medical book written by Fu Shan (傅山) in the 17th century and published in 1827, which discusses the diagnosis and treatment for disorders in obstetrics and gynecology.

came to my consultation room with her families. Her complexion was dark. She only uttered a few words before her tears rolled down her cheeks. With the help of her family members, I got to know the reason why she cried. She was pregnant soon after getting married. But she aborted the child because the couple didn't think they were ready to be parents. After a period of time, she was pregnant again, and this time she wanted to keep the baby. Unfortunately, she had a miscarriage two months later. Her third pregnancy attracted the attention of the whole family, including her husband, her parents-in-law, and her own parents, since all of them were afraid that she would have a miscarriage again. The woman also had a great pressure. Sadly, six months later, her fetus suddenly stopped growing. Since she was afraid that a recurrent miscarriage would happen, she came to me for consultation. It is clear that this patient was under great pressure. The treatment focused on the aspect of the liver. Medicinals were prescribed for her to soothe the liver, regulate liver *qi*, nourish blood, and regulate menstruation. Later, she gave birth to a healthy baby.

To sum up, pregnancy and menstruation are closely related to the liver. If women want to ensure normal menstruation and successful gestation, it is necessary to ensure the liver functions well with a good mood.

Q8. What is the relationship between breast diseases and the liver?

In addition to menstruation, breast development is the secondary sexual characteristic of women. Breasts secrete milk and provide vitality and power to raise offspring. They are important organs of women and symbols of feminine charm.

In modern society, an increasing number of people suffer from breast hyperplasia. A survey conducted by an institution in Shanghai showed that 77% of the white-collar women were diagnosed with breast hyperplasia in physical examinations, pointing out the fact that it is a common disease. Breast hyperplasia is called *ru pi* (乳癖 , meaning mammary lump) in TCM and has a close relationship with menstruation and emotional changes. According to *Huangdi's Inner Canon of Medicine*, breasts are mainly governed by the Stomach Meridian of Foot *Yang* Brightness. The Liver Meridian of Foot Reverting *Yin* goes through bilateral hypochondria, so the nipples are also in the charge of the liver meridian. TCM holds that breast diseases such as breast hyperplasia are closely linked to the liver meridian. Breast hyperplasia occurs due to the turbulent flow of *qi* and blood, leading to *qi* stagnation and blood stasis, which is associated with the liver and its meridian.

Breast hyperplasia has a close relationship with emotions which are supposed to be regulated by the liver. I once had such a patient in her thirties diagnosed with breast hyperplasia. She was very anxious. Her eyes went red when she was telling me about her disease. I asked why she had such a great pressure. She said that her living environment was very depressing. She lived together with her parents-in-law and frequently she had some arguments with them. She had hoped her husband could understand her. Contrarily, due to those conflicts, her husband gradually became estranged from her and they were on the verge of a divorce. From her account, it can be understood that she had been depressed and in a bad mood for a long time. This case illustrates that breast hyperplasia is closely related to mood. And it can be treated from the aspect of the liver.

To relieve breast hyperplasia, there is a patent medicine named Breast Lump Elimination Tablet (*rǔ kuài xiāo piàn* 乳块消片), once produced by the pharmaceutical factory affiliated to Beijing University of Chinese Medicine. It is quite popular as it is effective in the treatment for breast hyperplasia. The medicine contains Danshen Root, Szechwan Chinaberry Fruit (*chuān liàn zǐ* 川楝子), and Cow-herb Seed (*wáng bù liú xíng* 王不留行). These ingredients have the functions of soothing the liver, regulating *qi*, and promoting blood circulation.

Q9. What is the relationship between chloasma and the liver?

Some young female patients complain that it is not easy to be women. They say that after the child birth some marks and dark spots begin to appear on the face. One kind of spot typically occurs on the cheeks, some under the cheekbones and some right on the cheekbones without rising above the skin. It is light brown and called chloasma. It does not affect anything except appearance. But women love beauty and chloasma on the face is quite upsetting. They may try anything possible to get rid of it, including make-ups and laser treatment. Sometimes these methods are not effective and chloasma can be recurrent. So, they resort to herbal treatment.

Chloasma is a kind of skin disorder which does no harm to health. But you should not ignore it. TCM holds that there must be some root causes for the exterior manifestations. That is to say, the occurrence of chloasma may indicate you have some problems in your body if it is not due to the exposure to the sun. *Huangdi's Inner Canon of Medicine* suggests that it is related to the liver. 'Miraculous Pivot: Meridians' states that 'when *qi* in the liver meridian is disordered, one's complexion loses its luster, as if covered by a film of dust.' Therefore, chloasma is also called 'liver spot' in TCM. As was mentioned earlier, the liver can regulate the circulation of *qi* and blood. If it fails to function well or liver *qi* and blood are not sufficient to nourish the skin, chloasma may occur. Besides, the liver promotes *qi* movement, so if *qi* is stagnated, leading to blood stasis spilling over the skin, then chloasma develops. That is to say, chloasma can be caused by liver *qi* and blood failing to nourish the skin or by stasis of liver blood due to liver *qi* stagnation.

To prevent and treat chloasma, you should, first, keep a good mood; second, take some herbal medicine that can soothe the liver, regulate *qi*, and promote blood circulation; third, keep a good sleep schedule since sleep is the best cosmetic product.

Q10. What are the tips for women to boost mood?

To boost mood, women should protect the liver as the liver governs emotions. The liver is the basis for women's health. Characteristics of women, for instance, menstruation, menopause, emotional instability, and common diseases amongst women such as breast hyperplasia and chloasma are all related to the liver. Therefore, women should remember to always protect the liver, not only to boost mood, but also to preserve health and prevent disease.

Mood is so important that I have been emphasizing it in my lectures. There are some tips to lift your mood. You can tell yourself from time to time that no river is straight in this world and each river is winding. No highway is straight without a single bend. Life is like a river or a highway, which has twists and turns. There are ups and downs in life. So, you need to be optimistic.

To conclude, I'd like to highlight three points. First, smile more. Second, listen more. Third, talk more. These three tips may help you solve problems. Smiling can help you dispel anxiety, listening can help you build a bridge to communicate with others, and talking can help you release anger. Keep a good mood, and you will be healthy.

Chapter 10
Granary Officer: The Spleen

Q1. What is the spleen in TCM?

From the viewpoint of Western medicine, the spleen is an abdominal organ located in the left upper quadrant of the abdomen and below the left ribs in the human body while the liver is under the right ribs. It is involved in the production and removal of blood cells, forming part of the immune system. In contrast, the concept of the spleen in TCM is rather different. It is primarily involved in the transformation of food and drinks into blood and flesh. In other words, according to TCM, the spleen does not simply refer to the anatomical organ itself but the integration of part of the functions of the immune system, digestive system, nervous system, circulatory system, and many others in Western medicine.

A clinical case may illustrate such differences. A young man had his spleen removed in a surgery because of splenic rupture in a fight. After the splenectomy, however, he often felt generalized weakness, for which he visited a TCM doctor. The doctor observed his complexion and tongue and took his pulse after hearing his chief complaint. A diagnosis was made that he was suffering from spleen deficiency, which caused him feeling butterflies in his stomach. He thought to himself that his spleen deficiency probably could not be cured as his spleen had already been removed. He was so worried that he poured out his concern to the doctor. Breaking into laughter, the doctor comforted him explaining that the concept of the spleen in TCM is different from that in Western medicine. In a sense, splenectomy may affect some functions of certain systems, which may result in spleen deficiency, but the two are not the same. To be specific, the former does not necessarily cause the latter while the latter does not necessarily involve the former. Therefore, the TCM doctor told the young man: 'Now you happen to have had a spleen removal and spleen deficiency at the same time. But don't worry. I will prescribe you some herbal decoction that will probably make you better in a while.' The young man's symptoms were finally relieved.

In TCM, the spleen is often associated with the stomach. According to *Huangdi's Inner Canon of Medicine*, the two, like two brothers, are joined together by membranes and perform related functions. The stomach fulfills the function of receiving food. Chinese people sometimes ask each other a question whose literal translation is 'How is your stomach-mouth (*wèi kǒu* 胃口)?' In fact, they are talking about appetite, meaning 'Do you have a good appetite?' The stomach, like a pot, decomposes food. The spleen then plays a vital role in digesting it, transforming it into something useful and usable to the human body, and transporting the essence to the organs and tissues all over the body, turning it into blood and flesh. The spleen and the stomach are very important organs in humans as is well stated in 'Fundamental Questions: Secret Canon Stored in the Royal Library' that 'the spleen and the stomach are similar to a granary official and are responsible for digestion, absorption, and transportation of the five flavors.' In ancient times, granaries were storehouses for millet and rice. It is through the spleen and the stomach that the ingested food and drinks are turned into nutrients, so the two organs are often mentioned and studied together as the spleen-stomach or the 'spleen and stomach.'

Q2. Why is the spleen regarded as the postnatal foundation?

TCM believes that one has both prenatal and postnatal foundations, and one's lifespan depends on both. Only when one's prenatal and postnatal foundations are solid can one enjoy a long life.

How is one's prenatal basis formed? It comes from one's parents. As is mentioned in 'Miraculous Pivot: Life Span,' the human fetus is 'based on the mother's blood and defended by the father's essence' (*yǐ mǔ wéi jī, yǐ fù wéi shǔn* 以母为基，以父为楯). One interpretation is that the base of life is the *yin* blood of the mother, and the defense of life is the *yang* essence of the father, *shun* (楯) meaning railings literally. In Chinese rural areas, courtyards are often enclosed by wooden rails, which serve to protect one's home, marking the boundaries of one's territory. In this sense, 'defended by the father's essence' means the *yang* essence of the father protects the human body just like guard railings. Another interpretation is that the *yin* blood of the mother serves as the earth while the *yang* essence of the father is the seed, *shun* (楯) referring to the seed. In other words, the health of a fetus depends partly on the mother's *yin* blood and partly on the father's *yang* essence. Therefore, some people would take a pre-pregnancy test to find out whether the couple are in good health for making a strong baby because the parents' health status as the basis of prenatal foundation can affect that of the next generation.

To some degree, one's life span is determined by both prenatal and postnatal basis. It has been reported that many factors would affect the life span including social, environmental, geographic as well as hereditary factors, among which, however, lifestyle, also known as postnatal factors, plays a predominant role in deciding one's health status and lifespan. Among the postnatal factors, the spleen and stomach as well as the diet are especially significant.

Since ancient times, great importance has been attached to the spleen and stomach. According to 'Miraculous Pivot: Fasting in Healthy People' (*Líng Shū Píng Rén Jué Gǔ* 灵枢·平人绝谷), 'healthy people will die after seven days without eating food and drinking water.' The reasons are also explained in the *Canon*. A person's intestines and stomach can hold 3 *dou* (斗)[①] and 5 *sheng* (升) of food and water. Healthy people usually defecate twice a day, discharging 2.5 *sheng* of stool each time or 5 *sheng* in total each day. In a week they will discharge 35 *sheng* of stool, which is the total amount of food and water contained in the stomach and the intestines.

---

① *dou* (斗): measurement unit, 1 *dou* equals to 10 *sheng* or approximately 7.5 kilogram.

If all the food and water in the body has been completely discharged without any intake, people will die. Therefore, to determine whether a patient will live or not, physicians have to find out whether there is still food and water in the stomach and the intestines and whether one can still digest and transform them into essence or nutrients. Ancient Chinese people placed great emphasis on stomach *qi* as is written in 'Fundamental Questions: Pulse Conditions of Healthy People' (*Sù Wèn Píng Rén Qì Xiàng Lùn* 素问•平人气象论) that 'the loss of stomach *qi* is called adverseness which may lead to death.'

Q3. Why did ancient Chinese people value the spleen and stomach?

In terms of the five elements, the spleen and stomach pertain to earth, which is 'characterized by sowing and reaping' according to 'The Book of History: Great Principles' (*shàng shū hóng fàn* 尚书•洪范). To be specific, earth is closely related to sowing and reaping grain crops. Therefore, ancient Chinese people held that earth was of extreme importance to both the human body and the universe.

Shibo (史伯), a court historian during the reign of the King You of the Western Zhou dynasty (1046–771 BC), once remarked that emperors in ancient times created myriad things by mixing earth with wood, metal, water, and fire when he talked about the formation of the universe. The ancients meant to seek unity for everything in nature and regarded earth as the most fundamental element that formed myriad things. In the beginning, water was believed to be the most important element in 'The Book of History: Great Principles'. Then Shibo aired his view that earth was the most important one. In *Guan Zi*[1] (*Guǎn Zǐ* 管子), however, water regained the position of the origin of everything. As Zhang Liwen (张立文), a well-known professor of philosophy at Renmin University of China, has pointed out, this change over a period as long as 400 years reflected the transformation of the belief that

---

[1] *Guanzi*: an ancient Chinese political and philosophical text that was compiled around 475–221 BC and named for and traditionally attributed to Guan Zhong (管仲), the 7th century BC philosopher and statesman who served as the Prime Minister to Duke Huan of Qi (齐桓公).

the universe was constituted by some special elements, which was still a physical concept, into the belief that diverse natural phenomena could be unified with a philosophical concept. This philosophical concept finally centers on earth. Earth is therefore regarded as the postnatal basis that is particularly important to the human body.

Q4. How important are the spleen and the stomach to the human body?

To some degree, the spleen and the stomach can tell whether a severely ill patient can survive or not. A detailed explanation is available in *Huangdi's Inner Canon of Medicine*. According to 'Fundamental Questions: Genuine-*Zang* Pulses' (*Sù Wèn Yù Jī Zhēn Zàng Lùn* 素问•玉机真脏论), 'both the five excess conditions and the five deficient conditions can lead to death.' The five conditions of excess include forceful pulse, feverish skin, abdominal distension, difficulty in urination and defecation, and dysphoria and blurred vision, while the five conditions of deficiency include thin pulse, cold skin, shortness of breath, frequent discharge of urine and stool, and inability to intake food. The five conditions of excess refer to excess patterns in TCM resulting from the invasion of the five *zang*-organs by pathogenic factors. For instance, forceful pulse and difficulty in urination and defecation are manifestations of excess patterns. In the five conditions of deficiency, the five *zang*-organs become deficient due to deficiency patterns. Both types are critical conditions when the five *zang*-organs are attacked by pathogenic factors in the excess patterns and when they become deficient with insufficient essence in the deficiency patterns. That's why they will likely lead to death.

However, are there any exceptions? Yes. Also in 'Fundamental Questions: Genuine-*Zang* Pulses,' it is documented that after receiving treatment for a while, 'if one with deficiency patterns is able to have some rice porridge without frequent discharge of urine and stool, then one can be cured.' In other words, the *qi* of the spleen and stomach of the patient recovered since the patient no longer had loose stool after eating porridge. If patients with excess patterns could sweat a bit and defecate smoothly after having porridge, they could be cured as well because the pathogenic factors could be expelled by means of sweating and defecating. Of course, the *qi* of the spleen and stomach must be restored before the pathogens are expelled. The medication, assisted by the spleen-and-stomach *qi*, drives the pathogenic *qi* outside the body. It is evident that the spleen and the stomach are very crucial to the human body and the treatment of diseases. Similarly, in *Treatise on Cold Damage*[①] (*Shāng Hán Lùn* 伤寒论), one annotation is often written beneath many formulas, that is, sipping some warm thin porridge. For example, Cinnamon Twig Decoction (*Guì Zhī Tāng* 桂枝汤) is prescribed for common cold. After taking the medicine, the patient will be advised to have some warm thin porridge to preserve and promote the spleen-stomach *qi*, which is extremely important to the human body.

In the later generations, Li Dongyuan (李东垣)[②], one of the four great masters of TCM during the Jin and Yuan dynasties, wrote *Secrets from the Orchid Chamber*[③] (*Lán Shì Mì Cáng* 兰室秘藏) and *Treatise on the Spleen and Stomach*[④] (*Pí Wèi Lùn* 脾胃论) based on such descriptions of the spleen and stomach in *Huangdi's Inner Canon of Medicine* as was mentioned previously, resulting in the school of supplementing earth, which established the spleen's preeminence in both disease causation and as a focus of treatment.

In addition, when taking pulse at different places on the wrist, what is a TCM doctor looking for? The stomach *qi*, or vitality and root in pulse quality, is the top priority. *Huangdi's Inner Canon of Medicine* states that when stomach *qi* comes,

---

① *Treatise on Cold Damage*: a TCM treatise that was compiled by Zhang Zhongjing (张仲景) sometime before AD 220, at the end of the Han dynasty. It is amongst the oldest complete clinical textbooks in the world and considered one of the four canonical works of TCM.

② Li Dongyuan (李东垣): a famous Chinese medical expert and one of the four masters of Jin and Yuan dynasties in the history of TCM. As a representative of the school of 'invigorating the earth,' he founded the theory of the spleen and stomach. He and his theory of the spleen and stomach are valued by many doctors of later generations.

③ *Secrets from the Orchid Chamber*: a book on diseases of the spleen and stomach and many other clinical topics, providing 280 formulas in 28 categories.

④ *Treatise on the Spleen and Stomach*: one of the most important books in the history of TCM, in which Li Dongyuan lays the foundation for the elevation of the spleen and stomach as the postnatal root of *qi* and blood production.

the pulse is moderate and rhythmic. In other words, if the pulse of the patient feels moderate and smooth, there is stomach *qi*, which indicates that the ailment is curable.

Despite the slight differences in the pulse manifestations between the four seasons, that is, wiry and tight in spring while surging in summer, there should be stomach *qi* in the pulse. It is stressed time and again in the *Canon* that the patient can be cured when there is stomach *qi* and will die if there is none.

Q5. What makes the spleen the postnatal basis?

The spleen becomes the postnatal basis through its governance of transportation and transformation. In terms of TCM, transportation refers to the distribution of essence over the whole body, while transformation denotes change and digestion of food and water into blood and flesh. The two processes are governed by the spleen. According to TCM, the human body is a self-organizing holistic system. In 'Fundamental Questions: Significant Discussions on the Administration of Five Motions,' it is believed that 'transformation cannot be replaced by anything else.' The function of the spleen to turn the ingested food and water into blood and flesh is intrinsic to the human body and cannot be replaced by external forces. In this regard, TCM and Western medicine are quite different. To treat patients with blood insufficiency, blood transfusion is often adopted in Western medicine. However, in TCM, Angelica Decoction for Tonifying Blood is prescribed instead to supplement blood. It contains two major ingredients: Milkvetch Root and Chinese Angelica. Will the two ingredients generate blood when they are decocted? Never. The patient has to drink the decoction, which will be transformed and transported by the spleen before it acts on the *zang-fu* organs that generate blood in the human body itself. This is exactly the function of transformation carried out by the spleen, which cannot be replaced by anything external.

If such a function becomes insufficient, declines, or even fails, what will happen to the human body? The result will likely be fatal. 'Fundamental Questions: Soups and Liquors' states that patients whose 'spirit-*qi* does not work' may not survive. In this context, 'spirit-*qi*' means specifically the functions of digestion and distribution of the spleen and the stomach. Under normal circumstances, the medicine a patient takes is meant to act on some *zang-fu* organs to which one's spleen and stomach are supposed to transform and transport the medicine. When the spleen and the stomach fail to function properly, they are unable to take the medicine to where it is intended to act on, so the medicine the patient takes becomes useless. No matter what medicinals, food or water one takes, they cannot become something useful to the body when spirit-*qi* does not work, because of which the patient may face imminent death.

As was mentioned previously, the functions of the spleen and the stomach are closely associated with what people eat. However, due to some misunderstanding, people nowadays make some common mistakes. For instance, many people give the patients fruits as gifts. It is true that fruits are nutritious, but it is important to eat the right fruits at the right time. It is inappropriate to eat watermelon or banana due to the weakened digestive ability after a surgery. Since both fruits are cool in property, they may deteriorate the already weak functions of the spleen and stomach of the patient, hardly conducive to their recovery.

In pediatrics, there are recurrent fever cases due to malfunction of the spleen and stomach. Sometimes, when fever is just relieved in children, their parents are so loving that they would feed them for recovery with greasy food like fried chicken that they had regretfully missed during the fever. However, this would instead trigger their fever again. Why is that? The reason is explained in 'Fundamental Questions: Heat' (*Sù Wèn Rè Lùn* 素问·热论): 'Febrile disease tends to recur if meat is eaten when the disease is just alleviated, and heat may linger if excessive food is taken.' When the functions of the spleen and the stomach are weakened due to fever, neither meat nor a large amount of food could be digested, which, in addition to the remaining pathogenic factors, would cause fever to recur or be prolonged and make it difficult to cure.

Furthermore, the spleen transforms the water one drinks into bodily fluids and distributes them all over the body in addition to digesting, absorbing the food one takes in, and distributing the food essence. Clinically, there are also cases of nephritic edema. The patients' eyelids, face, and shanks are all swollen, especially the shins would become so swollen that a 'pit' or an indentation would appear and remain when pressed. In traditional Chinese medical terms, this is a pattern of excessive dampness due to deficiency in the spleen. Such diagnosis may confuse the patient: Why is nephritic edema in Western medicine a result of spleen deficiency in TCM rather than some kidney dysfunction? In fact, nephritis in Western medicine does not necessarily involve the kidney in TCM and the spleen in TCM is not equivalent to the kidney in Western medicine either. According to TCM, excessive dampness due to deficiency in the spleen refers to the condition where the water one drinks fails to be transformed into the body fluids or be distributed all over the body, and instead accumulates in some parts of the body symptomatically. The diagnosis is made in TCM based on the signs and symptoms. Therefore, 'Fundamental Questions: Significant Discussions on the Most Important and Abstruse Theory' states that 'all dampness diseases characterized by swelling and fullness are associated with the spleen,' as one of the nineteen items of pathogenesis. In other words, all symptoms of water retention due to excessive dampness are manifestations of the spleen's malfunction in water transformation and transportation.

Q6. What bodily functions does the spleen govern?

According to *Huangdi's Inner Canon of Medicine*, based on its transformation and transportation function, the spleen also fulfills two other functions. First, it governs blood. As the spleen governs transportation and transformation of food and drinks, much *qi* is generated in the process when food and drinks are transformed into nutrients. The *qi* enables the spleen to control blood. In daily life, some people suffer nosebleeds easily if their nose is bumped slightly. Some experience bleeding gums when they brush their teeth. Others bruise their arms and legs easily due to light bumps. In Western medicine, this is caused by low platelets. In TCM, however, it is attributed to spleen deficiency leading to insufficient *qi* that fails to contain blood.

Blood circulates in the body through the blood vessels which hold the blood. What governs the blood vessels? The heart. Additionally, the spleen secures and protects blood. Therefore, under the circumstances mentioned above, medicinal herbs that can reinforce the spleen could be prescribed such as Ginseng, Milkvetch Root, and White Atractylodes Rhizome. If spleen *qi* is reinforced, it can secure and protect blood, relieving the above-mentioned cases of bleeding.

Of course, in cases of nasal bleeding caused mainly by heat, heat should be cleared. The medicinals for reinforcing spleen *qi* are particularly effective for abnormal uterine bleeding due to *qi* deficiency, especially when menstrual periods are prolonged with large volumes of menses.

Second, the spleen governs the ascent of nutrients. Some people may feel general weakness or even fall asleep quickly after meals. One possible explanation is that blood concentrates in the spleen and the stomach after meals, unable to ascend to the brain and the heart, which is normal. On the other hand, in severe cases, the cause is spleen *qi* deficiency. Spleen *qi* fails to transport the nutrients upward to the head and the heart, resulting in general weakness, sleepiness, and lassitude. This disorder can be relieved with medicinals for strengthening and reinforcing the spleen.

Third, the spleen lifts the *zang-fu* organs and other body parts. Thanks to the gravity of the earth, *zang-fu* organs are pulled downward, but in a healthy human body, healthy *qi* would lift the *zang-fu* organs to its normal positions where they can perform their functions. It is the spleen that functions to prevent ptosis of *zang-fu* organs. It helps the *zang-fu* organs remain in their original positions as well as distributing the essence of the food and drinks outward and upward.

In cases of ptosis, '*qi* deficiency should be treated by lifting' according to 'Fundamental Questions: Significant Discussions on Phenomena Corresponding to *Yin* and *Yang*.' How? By supplementing and strengthening the spleen. The therapy is effective in cases of ptosis of the stomach and uterus and prolapse of the anus. Some patients suffer from uncontrollable drooping of the upper eyelids. What could help to lift the upper eyelid? The spleen and stomach. The upper eyelid fails to lift because of spleen *qi* deficiency which fails to govern the ascent of nutrients and to lift body parts. In such cases, Center-tonifying and *Qi*-replenishing Decoction should be prescribed to strengthen and harmonize the spleen and supplement *qi*.

Q7. How do you eat well to improve your spleen function?

The spleen, as the postnatal basis, governs transportation and transformation of food and drinks. It controls the blood and the ascent of nutrients and lifts the *zang-fu* organs and other body parts. Then what affects the spleen most? The diet. An appropriate diet is beneficial to your postnatal basis, the spleen and stomach. Poor diet, on the other hand, will give rise to spleen disorders. Chinese people are so much concerned with the diet that we greet each other with the question 'Have you had your meal?' Likewise, great importance is attached to the spleen and stomach.

You cannot be too careful with your diet given its close relation with the proper function of the spleen. In the process of evolution, many favorable dietary habits have been formed and should be preserved. For instance, seafood is often stir-fried with pepper or shredded ginger on the Shandong Peninsula, while it is often served with ginger juice and garlic in the city of Tianjin. As seafood is cold in property and ginger juice, garlic, pepper, and stir-frying are hot, the heat can offset the cold so that seafood becomes easy to digest.

In other places, seafood is fried, which could check its cool property. For the same reason, sashimi is eaten with mustard that is hot in nature. Some may argue that Westerners are different in this regard as they eat seafood served on ice with nothing else to savor the original flavor. But in fact, some Westerners may feel fine after eating seafood in such a way while others may suffer from vomiting and diarrhea. Therefore, good dietary habits should be observed.

Another example of proper dietary habit is the way people cook meat, especially greasy pork. When they stew pork in brown sauce, spices such as garlic, Chinese onion, ginger, Chinese cinnamon, and star anise are often added, which moves *qi* to relieve the greasiness of pork.

In Sichuan province where it is hot and humid, people enjoy hotpot in summer while they sweat heavily. The soup in the hotpot is covered with red chili pepper and Sichuan pepper, hence the reason for the name spicy hotpot. Others may wonder why they eat spicy food in such hot weather. That is because while it is humid in Sichuan, spicy food can remove dampness and move *qi*. According to TCM, the spleen likes dryness and dislikes dampness because the latter negatively affects the proper functioning of spleen *qi* whereas the former facilitates it.

Residents in some humid places, like balsam pear, which is bitter in flavor and dries dampness. According to 'Fundamental Questions: *Qi* in the *Zang*-Organs Following the Rules of Seasonal Changes' (*Sù Wèn Zàng Qì Fǎ Shí Lùn* 素问•藏气法时论), 'the spleen suffers from dampness which can be relieved by a bitter flavor'. In other words, food and medicinals bitter in flavor can be used to dry dampness to restore proper function of the spleen.

In Beijing, there is a tradition of eating pastry containing aged tangerine peel pungent and bitter in flavor and warm in nature. It dries dampness in the spleen. The above-mentioned dietary habits are all conducive to the function of the spleen, so they should be kept.

In terms of diet, *Huangdi's Inner Canon of Medicine* states that good dietary habits are key to health preservation. According to 'Fundamental Questions: Genuine *Qi* Endowed by Heaven in Remote Antiquity,' the sages in ancient times who knew the tenets for cultivating health followed the rules of *yin* and *yang* and adjusted their ways to cultivate health. They were moderate in eating and drinking.

To be moderate in eating and drinking means you should not eat or drink excessively and your diet should be regular. First, you should not overeat and should stop eating when you feel 70%–80% full. There are many causes of overeating. When enjoying buffet meals, it is likely that you will overeat to get the most out of it. Sometimes, when discussing business over meals with business partners, you tend to overeat because it often takes a long time. Another possible reason is that some people eat too fast to promptly register the brain's signal that they are full. In fact, after you start eating, it takes your brain at least 20 minutes to give you the signal that you are full. However, those who finish their meal within 20 minutes are likely to eat more than enough. Is overeating beneficial to the spleen and stomach, the postnatal basis? Absolutely not. In addition to stomach distention and stomachache, it may lead to obesity, high blood pressure, and heart disease. Therefore, I advise that you say no to overeating or overdrinking and be moderate in your diet.

Next, you should eat breakfast, lunch, and dinner at appropriate times regularly. Such dietary habits, a result of thousands of years of evolution, are reasonable enough for you to stick to.

One last piece of advice is that you should avoid eating food that is too hot or too cold. Some people like ice-cold food, which is very likely to impair your spleen-stomach function. The stomach, which is warm at the same temperature as that of the human body, that is, over 30°C, naturally does not welcome ice-cold food. Others may enjoy food at a high temperature such as the first couple of *jiaozi* (饺子 , dumpling) from a boiling pot. Such hot food will burn the esophagus and the stomach.

For the above reasons, Chinese ancestors stressed time and again that an appropriate diet is conducive to the spleen that serves as the postnatal basis, whose normal function will ensure normal life activities. So, you ought to protect your postnatal basis for better health.

Chapter 11

Magic Functions of the Spleen and Stomach

Q1. What role does the spleen play in the *qi* activity of the human body?

The spleen, the postnatal basis, governs transportation and transformation, transforming what people eat and drink into nutrients necessary for the human body. In addition, the spleen plays a pivotal role in the *qi* activity of the human body.

Sometimes when people, especially women, feel depressed, they would eat some sweets to relieve their symptoms of depression and lift their spirits. Since depression, or low spirits, is believed to be a manifestation of liver *qi* stagnation, why can sweets help relieve the problem to some extent? According to 'Fundamental Questions: Significant Discussions on Phenomena Corresponding to *Yin* and *Yang*,' 'pungent and sweet flavors function to disperse and pertain to *yang*.' In other words, food pungent or sweet in flavor disperses. As sweet flavors act on the spleen, the spleen distributes the nutrients sweet in flavor to the other *zang-fu* organs and all over the body. In this sense, sweet food can improve the function of the spleen, thus relieving liver depression. Its underlying rationale will be explained in detail in the following parts.

Q2. What is *qi* activity like in the *zang-fu* organs?

The *zang-fu* organs such as the heart, the lung, the liver, and the kidney in the human body seem motionless. This is not the case. *Huangdi's Inner Canon of Medicine* believes that there is constant *qi* activity in the *zang-fu* organs. That is to say, the human body is composed of *qi* that forms the *zang-fu* organs as well as other organs and tissues when it gathers. *Qi* is in constant movement. 'All diseases are caused by the disorder of *qi*,' according to 'Fundamental Questions: Pain' in *Huangdi's Inner Canon of Medicine*.

It is also believed that *qi* is constantly moving and changing in the body in many directions such as upward, downward, outward, and inward, or in other words, ascending, descending, exiting, and entering, hence the statement 'in all visible things, *qi* ascends, descends, exits, and enters' in 'Fundamental Questions: Significant Discussions on the Abstruseness of the Six Kinds of *Qi*' (*Sù Wèn Liù Wēi Zhǐ Dà Lùn* 素问•六微旨大论).

Since the heart and the lung are relatively high in position and the liver and the kidney are in lower positions, the ancient Chinese believed that *qi* of those in high positions should go downward while that of those in low positions upward, forming interactions and balance in terms of *qi* activity. In addition to descending, those in high positions also fulfill the function of dispersion. Take the heart as an example. It controls blood and vessels and corresponds to fire, which distributes and disperses. Meanwhile, heart fire should descend. The lung, in a high position, governs ventilation, distributing fine essence of food and water all over the body. According to 'Miraculous Pivot: Differentiation of *Qi*' (*Líng Shū Jué Qì* 灵枢•决气), 'the upper energizer initiates to spread the nutrients of food to all parts of the body... like the irrigation of dew and fog. That is what *qi* means.' The lung distributes nutrients like fog and dew downward from a higher position. It not only ventilates upward but also descends. Thanks to the lung, body fluids go downward. That is termed 'The lung oversees regulating the water passage.' One of the ways to treat retention of urine is to ventilate the lung just like removing the lid to pour water out of a teapot. Therefore, the lung performs both ascending and descending functions.

Similarly, both liver *qi* and kidney *qi* have the dual function of ascending and descending, distributing and gathering. Two points merit attention. First, *qi* is in constant movement and change in the *zang-fu* organs. As is believed in 'Fundamental Questions: Significant Discussions on the Abstruseness of the Six Kinds of *Qi*,' 'the mutual conditioning of generation and destruction emerges out of the movement of six *qi*. When there is unbending movement, changes occur.' In other words, *qi* is ascending, descending, exiting, and entering all the time in the human body including the *zang-fu* organs. That's why TCM doctors attach great importance to pattern differentiation and treatment. They would tailor the treatment to the development of disease. For instance, a prescription for tonification may be given to the patient one day and a prescription for purgation a couple of days later according to changes in signs and symptoms.

Second, human vital functions are made possible by the interaction between the heaven *qi* that descends and the earth *qi* that ascends. According to 'Fundamental Questions: Treasuring Life and Preserving Physical Appearance,' 'man exists thanks to the heaven *qi* and the earth *qi* and lives in accordance with the principle of the four seasons.' When the heaven *qi* and the earth *qi* fail to meet, people cannot enjoy normal vital functions. Therefore, it is stressed in 'Miraculous Pivot: Basic State of Spirit' that 'what the heaven has endowed man is virtue. What the earth has endowed man is *qi*. When the virtue and *qi* combine and communicate, life begins.' To be specific, the heaven provides people with sunlight, rain, dew, wind and so on and the earth minerals, plants, crops and so on, based on which human beings come into existence. Human beings' existence depends on the interaction between heaven and earth. In the human body, a mini universe that corresponds to nature, the *qi* activity in the *zang-fu* organs follows the same rule. The *qi* of the *zang-fu* organs in higher positions should descend while that of those in the lower positions should ascend so that the two can meet and communicate. Once they fail to meet because *qi* of those in higher positions moves upward and that of those in lower positions downward, the person may die soon.

It is documented in 'Fundamental Questions: Contraindication of Needling Therapy' that 'the liver is located on the left; the lung is stored on the right; the heart commands in the exterior; the kidney governs the interior.' Since the liver is in a lower position in the body, liver *qi* should ascend from the left side of the body. As the lung is in a higher position, lung *qi* should descend from the right side. According to 'Fundamental Questions: Significant Discussions on the Law of Motions and Changes of Original *Qi* in the Universe' (*Sù Wèn Tiān Yuán Jì Dà Lùn* 素问·天元纪大论), 'the left and the right are the routes for *yang* and *yin* to ascend and descend.' The ancient Chinese adopted a south facing orientation, so the left side is the east as the sun rises in the east and the right side is the west as the sun sets in the west. Therefore, they regarded left and right (east and west) as the routes of the ascending and descending of *yang* and *yin*. As the heart pertains to fire, it distributes *qi* from the interior outward and thus governs the exterior. The kidney, on the other hand, directs *qi* and blood inward from the exterior and thus governs the interior.

Q3. What role do the spleen and stomach play in the *qi* activity of the *zang-fu* organs?

Among the *zang-fu* organs, the spleen and stomach are of vital importance. Located in the center among the *zang-fu* organs, below the heart and the lung and above the liver and the kidney, the spleen fulfills the ascending function and the stomach the descending function. They are closely related to the ascending and descending functions of the other *zang-fu* organs. The *qi* of all the other *zang-fu* organs ascends when the spleen *qi* ascends and descends when the stomach *qi* descends. In this sense, the spleen and stomach are regarded as the pivot of the *qi* activity of the *zang-fu* organs and the human body. They play a mediating role among the *zang-fu* organs. 'The spleen serves for the other *zang-fu* organs; the stomach serves as a market,' as is described in 'Fundamental Questions: Contraindication of Needling Therapy.' A market is the place where exchanges of goods and various communication take place. The quote means the spleen and stomach work for the other *zang-fu* organs. According to *Hangdi's Inner Canon of Medicine*, the *qi* activity of the *zang-fu* organs is indeed regarded as an integrated whole, which reflects the holistic view of TCM.

This pivotal and mediating role of the spleen and stomach reminds me of a short-answer question in a previous test of clinical basics for doctoral program applicants of such specialties as Cold Damage, Golden Cabinet, and Warm Diseases. It went like this:

According to *Treatise on Cold Damage*, 'in Lesser *Yin* disease, there are signs and symptoms of diarrhea, sore throat, chest fullness, and vexation. Pig Skin Decoction (*Zhū Fū Tāng* 猪肤汤) can be used to treat it.' Why should the decoction be made aromatic during the decocting process?

The quotation can be analyzed in the following aspects. Lesser *Yin* refers to the Heart Meridian of Hand Lesser *Yin* and the Kidney Meridian of Foot Lesser *Yin*. Lessor *Yin* disease denotes the failure of normal physiological coordination between heart *yang* and kidney *yin*. The heart fire that is supposed to descend ascends instead while the kidney water that is supposed to ascend descends. As a result, sore throat and diarrhea occur. In addition, the heart fire that fails to descend gives rise to chest fullness and vexation. Therefore, Pig Skin Decoction is indicated to replenish the kidney water and reduce the heart fire. As for the question about the reason for making the decoction aromatic, some examinees answered simply that aromatic decoction tasted good and otherwise it would be unpleasant to take it. The answer was far from enough in such an examination related to *Huangdi's Inner Canon of Medicine*. The key is that the aromatic smell acts on the spleen to activate it. As the spleen and stomach play a pivotal role in the balanced function between the heart and the kidney, they were compared in ancient times to the matchmaker for mutual assistance and restriction between the kidney water and the heart fire. The spleen is also known as the yellow matchmaker because it corresponds to earth pertaining to the yellow color. Since water and fire are usually incompatible, a medium, that is, the spleen, is needed to coordinate them. This function of the spleen is extremely important.

The influence of the spleen and stomach over the ascending, descending, exiting, and entering functions of the *zang-fu* organs is based on the *qi* activity taking place in the organs themselves. The *qi* in an organ going upward does not mean it goes up only without going down. In fact, *qi* both ascends and descends in every organ. This corresponds to the theory that the function of one *zang*-organ is present in all the other four *zang*-organs just as one of the five elements is present in the rest four elements, embodying the holistic view in the *Canon*. That is why

Zhou Shenzhai (周 慎 斋), a TCM physician of the Ming dynasty (1368−1644), wrote in his book *Complete Medical Works by Zhou Shenzhai* (*Zhōu Shèn Zhāi Yī Xué Quán Shū* 周慎斋医学全书) that the spleen and stomach are present in every *zang*-organ. That is, there are the 'spleen and stomach' within the heart, the liver, the lung, the kidney, and even the spleen and stomach themselves. In other words, every *zang-fu* organ contains the spleen and stomach. There are two reasons to support this statement. First, the spleen is the postnatal basis that is contained in each organ. Second, the spleen and stomach serve as the pivot of *qi* activity, on which the ascending and descending functions of each organ depend.

A case in point is the well-known Six-ingredient Rehmannia Pill (*Liù Wèi Dì Huáng Wán* 六味地黄丸). Often prescribed to replenish kidney *yin*, it was first proposed in *Key to Diagnosis and Treatment of Children's Diseases* (*Xiǎo Ér Yào Zhèng Zhí Jué* 小儿药证直诀) by Qian Yi (钱乙) in the Song dynasty (960−1279). The main ingredients include three herbs for tonification and three herbs for purgation. The three reinforcing herbs are Prepared Rehmannia Root (*shú dì* 熟地), Common Yam Rhizome or Chinese Yam (*shān yào* 山药), and Asiatic Cornelian Cherry Fruit (*shān zhū yú* 山茱萸). The three purgative herbs are Poria Cocos, Water-plantain Rhizome (*zé xiè* 泽泻), and Tree Peony Bark. The reinforcing medicinals make *qi* ascend while the purgative ones descend. In a prescription for kidney deficiency, why are Indian Bread and Common Yam Rhizome included? As the two herbs act on the spleen and stomach, they enhance the ascending and descending functions of the spleen and stomach to promote and restore the functions of the kidney.

As mentioned previously, depressed people feel better after eating something sweet. The rationale behind it is now evident. Since the sweet flavor acts on the spleen, it improves the function of the spleen, conducive to the normal *qi* activity in all the organs and makes people happy. However, overconsumption of sweet food should be avoided. According to the *Canon*, one should not go to extremes and should stop using the potent medicinals when a disease is almost cured; otherwise, other diseases may arise. As for sweet food, it is emphasized in 'Fundamental Questions: The Interrelationship Between Life and Nature' that 'excessive intake of sweet flavors makes spleen *qi* stagnant and stomach *qi* thick.' This revised quote by later generations means if one eats too much sweet food, its stickiness will impede the spleen-and-stomach *qi*, leading to gastric and abdominal distension and poor appetite.

Q4. What will happen if the *qi* activity of the spleen and stomach is impeded?

For one thing, impeded *qi* activity of the spleen and stomach affects the spleen and stomach themselves, leading to digestive disorders. For another, it influences *qi* activity in the other *zang-fu* organs. Cases of the first situation are rather common. Failure of the spleen-and-stomach *qi* to ascend and descend properly will cause *qi* stagnation, which in turn results in blood stasis. Then patients will suffer stomachache, a result of the failure of spleen *qi* to ascend and stomach *qi* to descend, causing *qi* stagnation and blood stasis. Some would even turn pale and curl up in pain. In this case, the *qi* activity in the spleen and stomach should be regulated with potent traditional Chinese medicines such as Granules for *Qi*-stagnation Stomachache (*Qì Zhì Wèi Tòng Kē Lì* 气滞胃痛颗粒) available over the counter.

When stomach *qi* fails to descend, belching, hiccup and even vomiting will occur. Of course, sometimes, emetic therapy that involves vomiting is used to treat certain diseases. It is primarily indicated for pathogenic factors retained in the pharynx, esophagus, and chest, which causes severe sense of oppression. In such a case, emetic therapy can be prescribed according to the principle that 'if the pathogenic factors have accumulated in the upper position, vomiting therapy should be used' as is documented in 'Fundamental Questions: Significant Discussions on Phenomena Corresponding to *Yin* and *Yang*.' Since the pathogenic factors are in the upper position, it is reasonable to expel them from the above, that is, to vomit them out. There are many specific ways to induce vomiting including irritating the throat with a feather, drinking some salt water, and pushing a spoon, tongue depressor or even finger down to the throat over the tongue. However, this therapy should not be overused.

In addition, the failure of stomach *qi* to descend may lead to constipation, which is not uncommon clinically. It is referred to as turbid *yin* failing to descend, or abdominal fullness and distension according to the *Canon*. The most severe case I have encountered is a patient who had had no bowel movements for as long as 10 days, which was extremely distressing. Major Purgative Decoction (*Dà Chéng Qì Tāng* 大承气汤) is often used to address the problem. Its main ingredients such as Rhubarb (*dà huáng* 大黄), Sodium Sulfate (*máng xiāo* 芒硝), and Immature Orange Fruit can enable stomach *qi* to descend and in turn the turbid *yin* (urine and feces) to discharge. This therapy conforms to the descending trend of stomach *qi*. The most painful cases are those who feel the urge but have not enough strength to defecate. For such patients, medicinals for strengthening *qi* should be applied to give them the strength to defecate in addition to those that help stomach *qi* to descend.

While stomach *qi* should descend, the lucid *qi* (spleen *qi*) should ascend. If it fails to ascend, that is, 'if the lucid *qi* descends, it will cause diarrhea with undigested food in it' according to 'Fundamental Questions: Significant Discussions on Phenomena Corresponding to *Yin* and *Yang*.' Failure of the lucid *qi* to ascend can be attributed to deficiency. Therefore, treatment to invigorate the spleen and lift *qi* is often applied to patients with diarrhea.

The above therapy is frequently used in clinical practice. However, pattern differentiation should be the basic guiding principle. A patient of mine has had as many as five to six bowel movements every day for some 20 years. Many physicians would infer that such symptoms are probably the result of insufficient spleen *qi* that fails to ascend and lift, and thus medicinals for reinforcing *qi* and invigorating the spleen to lift *qi* should be prescribed. Unfortunately, such treatment proved ineffective for the patient. It then occurred to me that I should have asked about the quality of the feces in detail to make sure whether there was undigested food in it or whether it was sticky and difficult to flush away from the toilet. His reply was the latter, that is, his feces was sticky and odorous. Under such circumstances, the therapy of invigorating the spleen to lift *qi* is no longer applicable because stickiness indicates dampness heat. Instead, purgative medicinals to remove dampness heat in the large intestine was prescribed such as Chinese Pulsatilla Root (*bái tóu wēng* 白头翁), Ash Bark (*qín pí* 秦皮), Kudzuvine Root (*gě gēn* 葛根), Milkvetch Root, and Golden Thread. The outcome was quite satisfactory. This case warns the physicians that treatment should always be based on pattern differentiation rather than sweeping generalization.

People may believe that both stomach *qi* (turbid *yin*) failing to descend and spleen *qi* (lucid *qi*) failing to ascend are problems of the spleen and stomach themselves, affecting only their own functions. However, disorders of the spleen and stomach can affect the *qi* activity of the other *zang-fu* organs and give rise to a variety of diseases. Among them, insomnia and cough are two typical ailments.

Patients with insomnia suffer a lot. Some would toss and turn with eyes wide open for 2 or 3 hours trying to sleep in vain. Others do fall asleep but are very easily awakened sometimes only a couple of minutes after they close their eyes and are unable to fall asleep again. Some complain of dream-disturbed sleep. As sleep is regarded as a nutrient for normal mental activity, the lack of it makes people listless, causing anxiety, stress, and finally haggardness and mental fatigue.

According to *Huangdi's Inner Canon of Medicine*, *qi* circulates in the *yang* meridians in the human body in the daytime and *yin* meridians at night. Sleep is made possible when *qi* enters the *yin* meridians from the *yang* meridians at night. People feel sleepy and fall asleep thanks to normal *qi* activity as *qi* becomes peaceful in the *yin* meridians. When day breaks, *qi* enters the *yang* meridians from the *yin* meridians. Since *yang* corresponds to the exterior and activity, people wake up and begin to think and move around consciously.

If such normal *qi* activity is obstructed, that is, *qi* cannot enter the *yin* meridians from the *yang* meridians and remains in the latter, one's mind will be in an active state all the time and cannot fall asleep. By the same token, somnolence is also a result of impeded *qi* activity. When defense *qi* fails to enter the *yang* meridians from the *yin* meridians and is retained inside the *yin* meridians, one will feel drowsy because *yin* pertains to inactivity. One of my patients would fall asleep when riding a bike. He then fell into a ditch and continued to sleep there. This is caused by impeded flow of *qi*.

In *Huangdi's Inner Canon of Medicine*, it is believed that *qi* arrives at the *yin* meridians from the intestine and stomach meridians as the last leg of its journey in the *yang* meridians and arrives at the *yin* meridians from the spleen meridian as the last leg. Therefore, there is a saying that 'disharmony of the stomach disturbs sleep' according to 'Fundamental Questions: Disharmony.' In this context, the stomach refers to both the stomach and the spleen. The statement means that if the spleen and stomach fail to perform properly, the pivotal function in the *qi* activity of the *zang-fu* organs, or the *qi* flow in the *zang-fu* organs will be impeded. As *qi* cannot enter the *yang* meridians or *yin* meridians, somnolence and insomnia would occur. In the treatment, special attention should be paid to the pivotal role of the spleen and the stomach. A very effective formula was recorded in the Canon, that is, Pinellia Tuber and Broomcorn Millet Decoction. The ingredients, as the formula name suggests, are Pinellia Tuber and Broomcorn Millet. The decoction is said to be so effective that the patient would fall asleep as soon as they finish taking a whole dose. As a matter of fact, the two ingredients act to regulate the spleen and stomach and eliminate phlegm, restoring the ascending and descending functions of the spleen and stomach and *qi* movement in all the *zang-fu* organs.

Coughing is another symptom commonly encountered in clinical practice. For example, some patients suffer from coughs with profuse phlegm. Coughing seems to be most closely related to the lung, which controls *qi* and respiration. However, in 'Fundamental Questions: Cough' (*Sù Wèn Ké Lùn* 素问•咳论), it is believed that 'all kinds of cough are caused by accumulation of pathogenic factors in the stomach and are related to the lungs.' In other words, coughs indeed have something to do with lung disorders, but it is particularly closely related to the spleen and stomach. Therefore, there is another well-known statement about coughing in the same chapter of *Huangdi's Inner Canon of Medicine*, that is, 'The five *zang*-organs and the six *fu*-organs are all involved in coughing, not only the lung.' Therefore, in the treatment for coughing, physicians should not neglect the other *zang-fu* organs while treating the lung. All the *zang-fu* organs can affect the lung, giving rise to coughing. This is also an example of the holistic view advocated in the *Canon*.

The large amount of phlegm that accompanies coughing in some cases is due to the pathogenic factor that is accumulated in the stomach and related to the lung. According to TCM, the reason why phlegm comes into existence and cannot be transformed into normal body fluids lies partly in the spleen's dysfunction of transformation and transportation of water as was discussed in the previous chapter. When water fails to be turned into body fluids and distributed all over the body, some will transform into phlegm, which affects the lungs and results in productive coughing with phlegm. By now, a conclusion can be drawn. That is, to relieve coughs with phlegm, the ascending function of the spleen and the descending function of the stomach should be restored to resolve phlegm and eliminate dampness in addition to treating the lung because phlegm is a result of impeded *qi* activity in the spleen and stomach.

From the above, one can see that not only diseases of the spleen and stomach but also those of the other *zang-fu* organs are closely associated with the spleen and stomach because they play a pivoting role in the ascending and descending activity of *qi*. This understanding gives people the inspiration that the spleen and stomach should be treated when the treatment of directly affected *zang-fu* organs fails to yield positive results. Therefore, in 'Miraculous Pivot: Basic State of Spirit,' it is written that 'deficiency of spleen *qi* causes weakness of the four limbs and instability of the five *zang*-organs.' Based on this assumption, some prestigious TCM doctors such as Li Dongyuan proposed that all diseases should be treated from the perspective of the spleen and stomach. Such diseases include insomnia and coughing as discussed above, depression, stroke, hypertension, and cerebellar ataxia.

Mouth ulcers can also be treated from the aspect of the spleen and stomach. A male patient of mine suffered from ulcers in the tongue and mouth as well as private parts. In terms of Western medicine, he was diagnosed as having Behcet's syndrome. Treatments targeted at *yin* deficiency or *yang* deficiency failed to produce satisfactory outcomes. Eventually, he was treated with modified Ascending and Descending Powder (*Shēng Jiàng Sǎn* 升降散). Its main ingredients, including Stiff Silkorm (*jiāng cán* 僵蚕), Cicada Slough (*chán yī* 蝉衣), Wenyujin Concise Rhizome (*piàn jiāng huáng* 片姜黄), and Raw Rhubarb Root and Rhizome, act to regulate and facilitate the *qi* activities in the *zang-fu* organs especially the spleen and stomach. If the *qi* movement in the pivot (the spleen and stomach) becomes smooth, the other *zang-fu* organs are regulated to normal as well. To sum up, the argument that different diseases can be treated by regulating the spleen and stomach is based on their pivotal role in the *qi* activity of *zang-fu* organs. This is of significant clinical value.

Q5. What do you do to ensure proper function of the spleen and stomach?

Three points deserve attention if you would like to maintain proper function of the spleen and stomach.

First, diversify your diet in terms of the flavor or taste in the TCM sense. For instance, you should eat some food pungent and sweet in flavor. The reason is that these flavors are conducive to *qi* dissipation, which benefits the ascending of spleen *qi* and the descending of stomach *qi*; hence, it facilitates the pivotal functions of the spleen and stomach in the *qi* activity of all the *zang-fu* organs.

Second, avoid overeating. Do not eat too much at buffets or when it is other people's treat. Overeating impairs the spleen and stomach easily, leading to the failure of stomach *qi* to descend or spleen *qi* to ascend, which in turn causes myriad diseases. It is said that various diseases are caused by overconsumption of food and drinks, which should be taken with caution.

Third, have ease of mind. A feeling of wellbeing can help you stay away from stress, anxiety or feeling down. If chatting makes you feel better, chat away, which is good for health as I have mentioned in the previous chapters. If you enjoy singing, you can sing occasionally at a karaoke club or bar in your free time. According to TCM, singing acts on the spleen and helps spleen *qi* to ascend, which in turn coordinates the *qi* activity in the *zang-fu* organs all over the body. When the *qi* activity is smooth, you can have a good mood and health.

Chapter 12
Health Preservation of the Spleen and Stomach

Q1. What body parts and emotions are associated with the spleen?

According to *Huangdi's Inner Canon of Medicine*, man and nature are a union. Within this big union, there are five systems including wood, fire, earth, metal, and water. The spleen system, which comprises the spleen and stomach, pertains to the earth system. In addition to what are mentioned in Chapters 10 and 11, there are other aspects of the spleen-stomach system. For example, the spleen governs the muscles and the limbs. It opens into the mouth and manifests its splendor in the lips. It stores thoughts and the emotion that is most apt to affect it is overthinking.

Q2. What does it mean that the spleen governs the muscles and the limbs?

You might hear some people have had such an experience. A very strong, healthy, and energetic person can be wilting and spiritless after having experienced diarrhea for a few days. Just as the saying goes, even a strong man will become weak after having watery stools three times.

Some people may exhibit mental abnormalities such as climbing high to sing and taking off their clothes and walking. They present such great strength that it is hard to calm them down. Upon seeing these kinds of people, someone might suggest giving them certain purgative medicine. As is stated in 'Fundamental Questions: Manifestations of Diseases' (*Sù Wèn Bìng Tài Lùn* 素问·病能论), 'for those with anger and craziness... take away their food and they will be cured.' What does it mean to take away their food? Two explanations have been offered. One is to deprive the patient of the food, which is like hunger therapy as the modern treatment for mental diseases. Another is to remove the food in the stomach by inducing diarrhea or vomiting. Both diarrhea and vomiting make people weak. This is consistent with the belief that the spleen governs the muscles and the limbs.

According to 'Fundamental Questions: Greater *Yin* and *Yang* Brightness' (*Sù Wèn Tài Yīn Yáng Míng Lùn* 素问·太阴阳明论), 'the four limbs are nourished by stomach *qi*. But the latter is unable to reach their meridians directly. It is because of the spleen that the four limbs get their nourishment. When the spleen is diseased, it is unable to transport fluids for the stomach.' As a result, 'the four limbs cannot get nutrients and weaken day by day. The meridians become stagnant, and then the sinews, the bones, the muscles, and the flesh lose nourishment. Hence, the four limbs do not function.' In other words, when the nutrients of what one takes in can reach the muscles and the limbs, people will have strength. But in the case of diarrhea or vomiting, one is deprived of the nutrients of food and drinks. Hence, one will lack strength. Another point worthy of attention is that the stomach itself can't directly supply the nutrients for the muscles and the limbs. The nutrients can only reach the muscles and the limbs through the transformation-and-transportation function of the spleen. If the spleen and the stomach are in disorder, then the nutrients derived from what one eats can't reach the muscles and the limbs. Consequently, neither the muscles nor the limbs can get the nutritional supplement. That is why people have no strength.

If the muscles and the flesh don't get any supplies over a long period of time, one will weaken and become thinner day by day. Finally, symptoms may occur such as limb weakness, fatigue, shortness of breath, reluctance to talk, unwillingness to move and even muscle atrophy, which are categorized into atrophy-flaccidity syndrome. It is clearly stated in 'Fundamental Questions: Flaccidity' (*Sù Wèn Wěi Lùn* 素问•痿论) that 'to treat atrophy-flaccidity syndrome, select only the *yang* brightness' because the *yang*-brightness meridian is the sea of the five *zang*-organs and the six *fu*-organs and is responsible for moistening the ancestral sinew that controls bones and lubricates joints. In other words, the *yang*-brightness meridian is the source of *qi* and blood, and the *qi* and blood of *yang*-brightness meridian is indispensable to moistening the ancestral sinew. If the spleen and stomach are weak, especially when the spleen cannot transport and transform food essence, the muscles and the limbs will lose nourishment. Therefore, 'to treat atrophy-flaccidity, select only *yang* brightness.' Here, *yang* brightness refers to the spleen and stomach. *Huangdi's Inner Canon of Medicine* supplies a hint that physicians can treat the diseases of flaccidity and muscle wasting from the spleen-stomach aspect. Of course, those with *qi* deficiency should have *qi* replenished, and those with *yin* deficiency should have *yin* replenished.

There can be another pattern. The patient has dry stools and difficult bowel movements. In this case, tonic methods do not work. Instead, purgative therapy can help remove the dry stools and food accumulation so that the spleen and stomach can restore their normal functions. When the spleen and stomach can transport the essence of food and drinks to the muscles and the limbs, atrophy-flaccidity syndrome can also be alleviated. Therefore, for the treatment of atrophy-flaccidity syndrome, physicians should also make pattern differentiation before treatment.

Moreover, it is feasible for physicians to needle some acupoints in the spleen and stomach meridians, for example, *zu san li* (足三里 ST 36)[1] and *san yin jiao* (三阴交 SP 6)[2], to treat atrophy-flaccidity syndrome.

To sum up, if patients have muscle wasting and general weakness, physicians can treat them from the spleen aspect.

---

[1] *zu san li* (足三里 ST 36): an acupoint on the anteriolateral side of the leg, four-finger width under the kneecap, and outside the shin bone.

[2] *san yin jiao* (三阴交 SP 6): an acupoint on the medial side of the leg, four finger-width above the medial malleolus.

Q3. What food helps you build muscle?

According to 'Miraculous Pivot: Five Flavors' (*Líng Shū Wǔ Wèi* 灵枢·五味), for patients with a spleen disease, it is advisable for them to consume non-glutinous rice, beef, dates, and mallows. For those with a heart disease, they should consume wheat, mutton, apricots, and Longstamen Onion. For those with a kidney disease, they should consume black bean sprouts, pork, chestnuts, and bean leaves. For those with a liver disease, they should consume sesame, plums, and Chinese chives. For those with a lung disease, they should consume yellow millet, chicken meat, peaches, and scallions.

Huangdi's Inner Canon of Medicine proposes that different animal meats have a corresponding relationship with the internal organs of the human body. Specifically, pork corresponds to the kidney, mutton the heart, chicken meat the lung, lamb liver the liver, and beef the spleen. Those who practice bodybuilding or those athletes with weak muscles are often advised to eat beef because it contains rich amino acids that are used by muscles as the fuel. Consuming beef can supplement adenosine triphosphate good for muscle strengthening and growth. According to TCM, eating beef can help tonify the spleen. When spleen *qi* is tonified, it facilitates the transformation and transportation of the nutrients to the muscles and limbs. Hence, one builds strength and becomes strong.

Q4. What does it mean that the spleen governs the mouth and the lips?

In daily life, sometimes you may hear some people complain that whatever they eat is tasteless, with nothing tasting good. Others sometimes complain of a sweet taste and a sensation of greasiness in the mouth. Others still sometimes suffer from bitterness in the mouth. I once had a patient who reported that all he ate tasted like spiced peanuts. In fact, what he meant was he had bland taste or tastelessness in the mouth. Inspection shows that the lips of those patients, often, appear pale, dull, and far from full.

According to *Huangdi's Inner Canon of Medicine*, the spleen opens into the mouth (Fundamental Questions: Significant Discussions on Phenomena Corresponding to *Yin* and *Yang*). It manifests its splendor in the lips (Fundamental Questions: Six-Plus-Six System and the Manifestations of the Viscera). Moreover, it is clearly stated in 'Miraculous Pivot: Length of Meridians' that 'spleen *qi* passes through the mouth. When spleen *qi* is in harmony, one can distinguish the five flavors.' In other words, the spleen is believed to correspond to the mouth as each of the *zang*-organs has a corresponding orifice or opening in the head or face. Therefore, physicians can know whether the function of the spleen is normal or not by inquiring or by observing the patient's mouth. If one has a good appetite and a normal taste in the mouth, it means one's spleen functions well. If one feels tasteless in the mouth or has a sweet or a bitter taste in the mouth, it indicates there is a problem with the spleen and stomach. Some people may have accompanying symptoms including loss of appetite, mouth sores and ulcers. Physicians can also know whether the function of the spleen is normal or not by observing the lips of the patient. If the lips are full, ruddy, and lustrous, it means the functions of the spleen and stomach are normal. If the lips are dry and pale, it indicates there may be a problem with the spleen and stomach.

In fact, in the case of patients with a sweet taste and a sensation of greasiness in the mouth, they may have some existing lesions in the spleen and stomach. The disorder is named spleen-heat syndrome in 'Fundamental Questions: Strange Diseases' (*Sù Wèn Qí Bìng Lùn* 素问·奇病论), which means there is dampness heat in the spleen. According to the text, the spleen-heat syndrome is caused by frequent consumption of rich and greasy foods. If one often consumes sweet and fatty foods, indigestion may occur. Over time, internal dampness and heat can be generated, and spleen *qi* will move adversely upwards. Hence, one will develop spleen-heat syndrome, characterized by a sweet taste and a sensation of greasiness in the mouth.

For the treatment, Decoction of Fortune Eupatorium Herb (*Lán Cǎo Tāng* 兰草 汤) would be appropriate, which is one of the thirteen well-known prescriptions in the *Canon*. According to *Newly Revised Materia Medica* (*Běn Cǎo Cóng Xīn* 本草从 新) in the late Qing dynasty, people could wear Fortune Eupatorium Herb (*pèi lán* 佩兰) to ward off evil spirits, remove turbidity, and get rid of bad luck. As a chief ingredient in the formula, Fortune Eupatorium Herb is used to strengthen the spleen, drain dampness, and remove turbidity. In clinical practice, medicinals for removing heat such as Raw Gypsum (*shēng shí gāo* 生石膏), Common Anemarrhena Rhizome (*zhī mǔ* 知母), Divaricate Saposhnikovia Root (*fáng fēng* 防风), Agastache (*huò xiāng* 藿香), and Poria Cocos are usually added to help treat spleen-heat syndrome with a sweet taste in the mouth. Often, good results can be obtained.

With the improvement of living standards, it is likely that people often eat well and feel full. Then the rate of incidence for bad breath is also on the increase because of the dampness heat in the spleen and stomach and indigestion. When you suffer from halitosis, you will feel embarrassed and have to cover your mouth when speaking to others.

To get rid of bad breath, you can take the Decoction of Fortune Eupatorium Herb. To prevent it, you can eat some hawthorns, turnips, and sweet potatoes.

First, consume hawthorns to promote digestion and resolve food stagnation. Hawthorn is believed to have the function of removing stagnation and food retention. You can eat some hawthorns to help digestion. In addition, any experienced cook knows that meat can be quickly boiled soft by adding several hawthorns to the stewpot so that it will be easy to eat and digest.

Second, consume turnips to remove gastrointestinal heat. TCM believes that turnips are good to human health. They can remove the dry heat and clear stagnant *qi* from the body. Their cooling effects are especially beneficial to the digestive system and can result in an increase in *qi* circulation so that bad breath can be relieved. Zheng Banqiao, one of the eight eccentricities in Yangzhou, Jiangsu province and a well-known calligrapher and a painter of the Qing dynasty, once created a couplet telling the secret of health preservation. It reads: 'Greens, turnips, and brown rice; a pot of chrysanthemum tea is nice.'

Third, consume sweet potatoes to improve bowel movements. People with unpleasant breath are usually found to have problems with defecation. Sweet potatoes contain high fiber content and thus can stimulate bowel movements and help relieve bad breath. The fact that it becomes a well-known food to relieve constipation is related to an emperor in the Qing dynasty.

As you may know, Emperor Qianlong (1711-1799) lived up to 87 years old, which made him the longest living emperor of China. In his later years, he developed constipation, and many prescriptions failed to alleviate it. One day, he wandered to the imperial kitchen and smelled a very sweet scent. Qianlong was curious and asked the servant what it was. The servant told him that it was the baked sweet potato, usually eaten by the servants or the poor people. The emperor had never eaten it before. Its good smell made Qianlong long for a taste. So, he asked for the baked sweet potato for a try. Breaking it off and tasting it, he found it delicious and had liked the baked sweet potato ever since. He often ordered baked sweet potatoes or sweet potato porridge. Over time, his constipation was relieved. Hence, sweet potato became well-known. Today, it is believed to be a food with crude fiber that facilitates bowel movements. So, those with bad breath can eat some sweet potatoes to relieve the symptoms. But those with a weak spleen and stomach should take caution to avoid overconsumption. In addition, TCM believes that sweet potato can harmonize blood, tonify *qi*, and replenish the five *zang*-organs.

Q5. What does it mean that the spleen governs drool?

The spleen opens into the mouth. Some people have excessive saliva in their mouth, which causes drooling problems. According to TCM, drooling is a symptom of spleen disorder.

I once treated a patient who found himself with a lot of saliva in his mouth when he got up in the morning. He therefore had to frequently spit it out, thin and white. To treat this kind of disorder, regulating the spleen and stomach is the key. TCM believes that the spleen and stomach govern the transformation and transportation of not only the essence of food and drinks but also the fluids. If spleen *qi* is unable to transform the fluids and tangible water develops, then saliva would come from the mouth. Therefore, for such patients with drooling problems, physicians should replenish their spleen-stomach *qi* and warm their spleen *yang*.

To relieve drooling, treatment based on pattern differentiation is of pivotal importance. Some patients have thin and white saliva, while others may have yellow and thick saliva. Still others may have drool stains on their clothes. For the latter two, physicians cannot warm their spleen *yang*. Instead, spleen heat should be removed. That is, physicians should distinguish cold and heat patterns before prescribing medicinals.

Those who drool at night are also likely to suffer from some problems in the spleen and stomach and are advised to seek medical consultation.

You may find some children love to blow bubbles with their saliva. Some people regard it as a sign that their teeth are beginning to emerge. According to TCM, this can be a manifestation of excess saliva, which indicates that there may be a minor problem with the spleen and stomach of the child. It is thus advised to use some children's medicine to eliminate food stagnation and strengthen the spleen.

For those who are too young to take medicine, you may give them a massage by tonifying the five meridians. Each of the five fingers corresponds to the meridian of a particular *zang*-organ. For example, the thumb corresponds to the spleen meridian; the index finger, the liver meridian; the middle finger, the heart meridian; the ring finger, the lung meridian; and the little finger, the kidney meridian. So, to tonify the spleen meridian, you may stroke from the tip of the thumb to its root of the baby for about 500 times, which can be beneficial to strengthening the spleen. (See Figure 12-1)

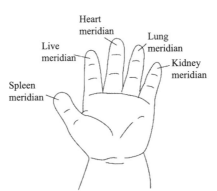

Figure 12-1   Tonifying the five meridians

There are other massage techniques to boost your child's digestive functions. First, you can rub your child's abdomen quickly and lightly in a clockwise direction around his navel. Second, you can use spine pinching. You put your fingers on each side of the base of your child's spine, pinch and roll the skin upwards till the base of the neck and repeat it for a couple of times. Third, you can knead the acupoint of *zu san li* on the outer calf of your child, which is also very beneficial to the digestive system. (See Figure 12-2, Figure 12-3 and Figure 12-4)

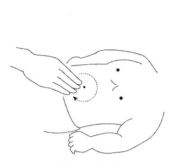 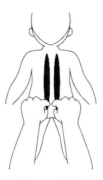 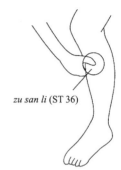

zu san li (ST 36)

Figure 12-2	Figure 12-3	Figure 12-4
Abdomen rubbing	Spine pinching	Kneading *zu san li* acupoint

Q6. What does it mean that the spleen manifests its splendor in the lips?

TCM believes that the lips are dominated by the spleen. That is, if the spleen and stomach function well, *qi* and blood will be sufficient, and the lips will be ruddy and lustrous. Nowadays, some girls live an irregular life. They often stay up late, sometimes eat too much and sometimes skip or neglect their meals. Over time, these bad living habits may cause the disharmony of the spleen and stomach. If so, how do they expect to have ruddy and beautiful lips? Some girls resort to expensive cosmetics, painting their lips with lipsticks. Isn't this putting the cart before the horse? The right thing to do is balancing work and leisure time to restore regular life. In this way, the lips can be nourished by the essence of food and drinks. Naturally, they can be full, plump, lustrous, and gorgeous.

Q7. What does it mean that the spleen governs overthinking?

Overthinking is a term that includes thinking, imaginations, intentions, and some of the ideas that one produces.

Thinking is good and positive, but if one spends a long time figuring something out or dwelling on something, one's spleen *qi* might be impaired, bringing about dysfunction of the spleen. In the Jin dynasty, there was a doctor named Zhang Zihe (张子和) who wrote a famous book called *Confucians' Duties to Their Parents* (*Rú Mén Shì Qīn* 儒门事亲). In the book he documented how he treated a woman who suffered from overthinking. The woman was preoccupied with family issues and overthinking took away her appetite. She grew thinner day by day and finally suffered from insomnia. Her father had consulted many famous doctors for treatment, but all had failed to cure her in the past two years. Finally, Zhang Zihe was invited. He offered an idea to the woman's father. After obtaining the agreement, Zhang Zihe then went to their home to drink and eat, and asked for consultation fees, but he didn't treat the woman at all. The same thing repeated for several days. The woman became so angry that she even perspired. After profuse sweating, she was able to fall asleep right that night.

Overthinking can cause *qi* binding. When *qi* binds, it is unable to flow freely and thus causes spleen dysfunction. As a result, the woman had no appetite at all. When the woman didn't take in any food, no nutrients could be absorbed by her body, and she lost weight. In this case, Zhang Zihe used the method of one emotion conquering another. To be specific, anger can conquer overthinking. Anger is governed by the liver which corresponds to the element of wood. Wood can restrict earth, to which the spleen pertains. When the woman got furious, *qi* and blood flew adversely upwards and removed the stagnation caused by overthinking.

Since overthinking may cause impairment to the spleen, it is advised that one should not split hairs but be optimistic and try looking at the bright side of the things.

According to 'Miraculous Pivot: Basic State of Spirit,' 'the spleen stores nutrient *qi* and nutrient *qi* houses intentions.' Those who think too much or are overly outspoken may have a spleen disorder. The latter is termed 'the spleen failing to house intentions.' Here is a medical case to illustrate it.

A few years ago, I followed my mentor Prof. Wang Hongtu to practice medicine. One day we came across a 17-year-old girl, who was diagnosed with adolescent schizophrenia at some psychiatric hospitals. She was restless with auditory and tactile hallucinations and presented illogical reasoning. Moreover, she loved singing and was always humming, whether it is a high-pitched or low-pitched song. Besides, she expressed her like for the opposite sex in a conspicuous manner. When her brother's male classmates came to their home, she would offer them tea and cigarettes. When the female classmates came, she would refuse to come out of her room, let alone talk to them. She often pictured in her mind having contact with the opposite sex. She said that she preferred to be with boys and always wanted to sing.

At the beginning, we thought she had dampness heat in her liver and gallbladder, so Prof. Wang Hongtu treated her from the perspective of clearing heat and purging ministerial fire in the liver and the gallbladder. After some treatments, the symptoms of restlessness and auditory and tactile hallucinations were relieved. However, her desire to sing and to contact the opposite sex was not alleviated. Later, Prof. Wang thought of the statement in *Huangdi's Inner Canon of Medicine*: 'The spleen stores nutrient *qi* and nutrient *qi* houses intentions.' The girl always wanted to expose her ideas and intentions—this is the result of the spleen failing to house intentions. The spleen was disturbed by heat, resulting in the failure of the spleen to keep intentions to herself so that what she thought was exposed. Therefore, the herbal formula was changed into Spleen-Purging Powder (*Xiè Huáng Săn* 泻黄散) which contains only a few medicinals such as Agastache, Cape-Jasmine Fruit, Gypsum, Divaricate Saposhnikovia Root, and Licorice. On this basis, the formula was modified in accordance with manifested signs and symptoms. Three months later, her condition was finally controlled.

Don't get me wrong. It is advised that those who feel depressed should sing songs to vent emotions. But if one always feels like singing, one might have spleen disorder as singing pertains to the spleen among the five voices[1].

Q8. What is the relationship between the spleen and seasons?

The human body and nature form a unity, and the *zang-fu* organs and seasons

---

[1] five voices: referring to shouting, laughing, singing, crying, and moaning; they respectively pertain to the liver, the heart, the spleen, the lung, and the kidney.

constitute a unity. It is repeatedly stated in *Huangdi's Inner Canon of Medicine* that a particular organ corresponds to a particular season. For instance, the liver is related to spring, the heart to summer, the lung to autumn, and the kidney to winter. The spleen, nevertheless, is special, for which there are two versions of the relationship between the spleen and seasons. The first one is that the spleen governs late summer. The second one is that the spleen doesn't rule a specific season by itself. Instead, the spleen rules the four seasons. These two viewpoints originate from different pairings with the five elements. That is, the two sayings discuss the intimate relationship between the spleen and seasons from different perspectives.

Let's start with the first saying: the spleen governs late summer. Late summer is called *chang xia* (长夏, literally long summer) in Chinese and refers to the last month of the lunar calendar, usually between mid-July and August. It is also called *ji xia* (季夏) in *Huangdi's Inner Canon of Medicine*. The late-summer season is characterized by both heat and dampness (plenty of rainwater). The most likely product of the mutual steaming of heat and dampness is transformation. For example, food undergoes the most rapid change in late summer. If you put a bowl of rice in a humid environment, it will be fine in the morning, but at noon its color changes. In an even hotter place, it may turn yellow in the afternoon due to fermentation. There are changes in the food, which means qualities are changed and new things are generated. Therefore, it can be said that transformation is closely related to high temperature and steaming of dampness heat.

Likewise, the spleen governs transformation of food and drinks. It likes dryness and is intolerant of dampness. It is also responsible for transforming and transporting fluids. The failure to do that causes fluid retention and is attributed to the spleen. Therefore, the characteristics of the spleen match the characteristics of the late-summer season. So late summer corresponds to the spleen. This is what it means: the spleen governs late summer.

In summer, you likely have epigastric distension and loss of appetite due to dampness heat. To relieve them, you'd best take something to strengthen the spleen and dry dampness. For example, eating barley rice porridge, Poria Cocos cakes or Tangerine Peel cakes is conducive to strengthening the spleen and removing dampness, and is good for you to increase appetite. Some people may prefer drinking mung bean soup to relieve summer heat, which is also a good choice.

Now let's look at the second saying: the spleen doesn't rule a specific season by itself. It is stated in *Huangdi's Inner Canon of Medicine* that the spleen pertains to earth. The earth produces myriad things and follows the law of heaven and earth. Zhang Jiebin (a well-known physician of the Ming dynasty) also stated: 'Earth is the basis of everything. The spleen-stomach is the basis of the *zang-fu* organs. So, it can nourish from head to toe in each season. How can it unilaterally rule a specific season by itself?' In other words, the spleen nourishes people from head to toe with the essence of food and drinks from the spleen and stomach. Besides, the spleen doesn't rule a specific season. Spleen *qi* exists in all seasons throughout the year as the spleen pertains to earth and is in the center among the *zang-fu* organs. Earth is regarded as the mother of all living things, and the spleen and stomach provide the material basis of the acquired constitution. The spleen nourishes everything just like earth nurtures myriad things.

In previous chapters, I mentioned that Shibo, the imperial court historian of King You of the Western Zhou dynasty, proposed that earth mixed with wood, fire, metal, and water should generate myriad things. Therefore, you should always maintain the health of your spleen and stomach throughout the year because they are the foundation. That is why in many herbal formulas, there are some herbs specially prescribed to strengthen and guard the spleen and stomach. *Treatise on Cold Damage* contains quite a few formulas that require you to drink hot thin porridge after taking herbal medicine, aiming to protect the spleen and stomach.

Q9. How do you preserve the health of the spleen and stomach?

The spleen and stomach are the foundation of acquired constitution, which is very important for human health. To maintain spleen-stomach health, you should keep in mind the following points.

First, you should balance your diet, avoid overeating, and stay away from greasy foods. Remember to eat your meals regularly and make sure the meals are of mild temperature, neither too hot nor too cold. Don't eat too much as it is repeatedly stressed in *Huangdi's Inner Canon of Medicine* that illness originates from overconsumption.

Second, you should pay attention to the characteristics of the spleen, that is, the spleen likes dryness and is intolerant of dampness. Accordingly, you should mind your diet. You may eat some foods that are spicy or bitter in taste. Spicy and bitter foods along with foods mild in nature can help relieve dampness. You are advised to consume some peppers, chilies, and balsam pears. In addition, Poria Cocos and Dried Tangerine Peel are also good to remove dampness.

Third, you can get some acupoint massages to strengthen the spleen and stomach. One of the recommended acupoints is *zu san li*, which belongs to the Stomach Meridian of Foot *Yang* Brightness. It is on the anteriolateral side of your lower leg, four finger width under your kneecap, and outside your shin bone. Another point is *san yin jiao* of the spleen meridian. It is on the inner side of your lower leg, three *cun* (four finger width) above your medial malleolus. Often kneading these two acupoints is helpful to the spleen-stomach function. (See Figure 12-5)

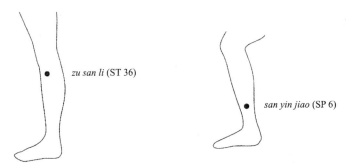

Figure 12-5   *Zu san li* acupoint (lateral) and *san yin jiao* acupoint (medial)

Finally, you should avoid overthinking. Remember that no river in the world is without a turn. No road in the world is without a curve. The same is true with your life. There might be twists and turns, and you may have some rough experiences. You should be open-minded and avoid thinking too much.

Chapter 13
Prime Minister: The Lung

Q1. What does the first cry of the newborn tell you?

As is known to all, a newborn baby comes into the world with a cry. This first cry is regarded as the most beautiful sound in the world. It signifies the birth of a little human being. Some people may raise questions and wonder why the newborn baby cries as soon as he/she is born.

Among the seven emotions of TCM including joy, anger, anxiety, overthinking, sorrow, fear, and fright, only joy is the real positive emotion. The remaining emotions are either neutral or negative. The newborn baby may sense that he/she will come to this world with a life of ups and downs. Maybe the baby does not want to come to this world, so he/she cries as soon as he/she is born. Other people think that when a baby is born, he/she leaves the womb and feels scared. The newborn has a good reason to cry because of the sudden entry into a strange and cold world after having been in a warm comforting place for ten months. Therefore, the baby is terrified and cries. Is this the case? Some newborn babies do not cry after birth, and doctors have to lift their legs and pat their bottoms to make them cry.

What does a newborn baby's first cry really mean? In fact, it signals the first time that the newborn must use his/her own lungs to breathe. From then, this spontaneous breathing has been established, and so has the pulmonary circulatory system. It signifies that this individual, the newborn, can live independently in this world and no longer depends on the mother for oxygen. Before a baby is born, he/she must take in oxygen from the placenta through the umbilical cord. Now he/she is breathing clear air in nature on his/her own to maintain life.

The lungs, responsible for breathing, play a very critical role in one's vital functions. Breathing marks the beginning of life. If breathing stops, it means the end of life. As a result, *Huangdi's Inner Canon of Medicine* attaches great importance to the lung. (Please note that the singular form is used when we refer to the concept of the lung in TCM.)

Q2. How does TCM describe the lung?

According to Western medicine, the lungs (the left and the right) are in the chest. They are connected to respiratory tract, nasal cavity and pharynx, and exchange gasses with natural clean air. According to TCM, as is stated in 'Fundamental Questions: Manifestations of Diseases,' 'the lung is the canopy of the *zang*-organs' because it is in a higher location. The canopy refers to the umbrella-shaped cover placed above a carriage seat in which the monarch or emperor sits. The lung is above the heart, which is like the canopy over the monarch or emperor.

Q3. What is the role of the lung?

Huangdi's Inner Canon of Medicine gives an official title to each of the *zang*-organs. For example, 'the heart is the monarch,' according to 'Fundamental Questions: Secret Canon Stored in the Royal Library.' The liver is the general of the whole nation. The spleen and the stomach are the granary officers, who function like a support system for logistical operations. The lung is the organ to assist the heart, which is like *xiang fu* (相傅 prime minister) to assist the monarch. *Xiang* (相) is the head of civil officials, like *cheng xiang* (丞相) or *zai xiang* (宰相) in ancient

China. Some well-known historical figures, like Zhuge Liang, Li Si (李 斯)^① and Xiao He (萧何)^② had served as the prime minister in their times. The prime minister is only second to the emperor and governs the whole country, so you can understand how important he is.

In *Huangdi's Inner Canon of Medicine*, the lung is compared to the prime minister of a country. As you can imagine, the functions of the lung are enormously great. As 'Fundamental Questions: Secret Canon Stored in the Royal Library' reads, 'the lung is the organ like a prime minister and is responsible for management and regulation.' That is to say, the lung takes charge of regulating the functions of the other *zang*-organs. The spleen produces nutritive substances and gives them to the lung. Then the lung is responsible for distributing the nutrients to various *zang*-organs. It determines the amount that is allocated. In fact, the lung maintains the normal functions of all *zang-fu* organs, and thus oversees the general condition of the whole body.

Q4. What are the physiological functions of the lung?

There are mainly four functions. First, the lung governs breathing and *qi*. Second, the lung governs diffusion, dispersion, depuration, and descent. Third, all meridians and vessels converge in the lung. Fourth, the lung governs regulation of water passage.

Q5. What does it mean that the lung governs breathing and *qi*?

The lung controls breathing and governs *qi*. At the mention of physiological functions of the lung, you know intuitively that the lung connects the airway, throat, and nose. Hence the lung controls breathing and connects the human body with

---

①   Li Si (李斯): Prime Minister of the Qin dynasty (221–206 BC).

②   Xiao He (萧何): Prime Minister of the Western Han dynasty.

nature as a whole. This understanding of the lung is the same as what Western medicine explains. In addition, *Huangdi's Inner Canon of Medicine* believes that the lung governs *qi*, which is a bit different from the understanding of Western medicine doctors. It contains two levels of meaning: the lung governs respiratory *qi* and *qi* in the whole body.

First, the lung governs respiratory *qi*. That is what we call the process of gas exchange between the human body and nature, which is controlled by the lung. We inhale the clear air from nature, take in the nutritious substances and deliver nutritious clear *qi* to all parts of the body. Meanwhile, we exhale turbid *qi* (carbon dioxide). According to 'Fundamental Questions: Significant Discussions on Phenomena Corresponding to *Yin* and *Yang*,' 'heaven-*qi* communicates with the lung.' If we have trouble breathing and have lung problems, then symptoms of cough, asthma and even hypoxia may occur. Therefore, it is clearly stated in 'Fundamental Questions: *Qi* in the *Zang*-organs Following the Rules of Seasonal Changes' that lung diseases first affect respiratory function. It reads: 'Lung diseases are characterized by panting, coughing, and adverse flow of *qi*.'

I once treated an old lady over 80 years old, who coughed all night long. One of her family members told me that every night she coughed out thin white phlegm that filled two plastic bags. The old lady was very weak, with tightness in her chest and shortness of breath. She would be out of breath after walking a few steps, let alone stair climbing—she wasn't able to climb stairs at all. This disease was treated from the lung aspect. She was given herbs to sooth and strengthen her lung to breath. Phlegm-dissolving medicinals were also prescribed to reduce her phlegm. She was finally cured.

In the medical case I mentioned above, the patient had symptoms of shortness of breath and chest tightness besides cough and asthma. In other words, she lacked strength, but why is that? That is the second level of meaning: the lung governs *qi* in the whole body. 'Fundamental Questions: Six-Plus-Six System and the Manifestations of the Viscera' states: 'The lung is the root of *qi*.' Here, *qi* refers to the *qi* in the whole body. There are a few Chinese idiomatic expressions containing the *qi* to describe people such as *qi yu xuan ang* (气宇轩昂, having an imposing appearance), *xue qi fang gang* (血气方刚, being impetuous and easily given to passions), and *shen qing qi shuang* (神清气爽, being refreshed and invigorated). The *qi* in the whole body consists of two aspects: 1) nutrients transformed from the essence of absorbed food and drinks; and 2) the fresh air that the lungs absorb.

Q6. What is pectoral *qi*?

Pectoral *qi* is the combination of the fresh air inhaled by the lung with the essential *qi* from the nutrients of food and drinks transformed and transported by the spleen and the stomach. It forms in the chest and is controlled by the lung, assisting the heart in promoting blood circulation. It is also the force for respiration, voice, and body movements. If a person's voice is loud, it can be said that the pectoral *qi* of this person is sufficient. If the voice is low and weak and somewhat hoarse, pectoral *qi* is insufficient or sinking.

Another function of pectoral *qi* is that it permeates the heart and the vessels. The vessels are governed by the heart, which means every vessel has connections with the heart. Pectoral *qi* can travel through the heart vessels to promote blood circulation and *qi* movement. Hence, 'Miraculous Pivot: Pathogenic Invasion' states: 'Pectoral *qi* accumulates in the chest, runs up to the throat, penetrates through the heart vessels, and drives respiration.'

Q7. What does it mean that the lung governs diffusion, dispersion, depuration, and descent?

The second major function of the lung is that, according to TCM, the lung governs not only diffusion and dispersion, but also depuration and descent. The two aspects cooperate and should be in harmony.

I want to talk about a phenomenon. We all have cell phones, but how can cell phones receive text messages? It relies on signal coverage. You can see that the cell tower is usually built very high to achieve wider coverage. It is only within the mobile coverage zone that your cell phone can receive text messages. The same is true of the human body. To distribute the nutritious substances to all *zang*-organs, the lung should take a high position. So, the lung is located at the top of all *zang*-organs, which is called the canopy.

'Miraculous Pivot: Differentiation of *Qi*' describes this function as 'the upper energizer initiates to distribute the nutrients of food to all parts of the body to steam the skin, fill the body, and moisten the hair in the same way as dew and fog provides humidity. That is what *qi* means.' Here, please note the expression that 'the upper energizer initiates to distribute' refers to the lung with its function of diffusion and dispersion. Therefore, the nutrients of food and drinks can be diffused and dispersed to the whole body like fog and dew. The *qi* not only consists of the nutrients derived from food and drinks, but also fresh air from nature. As for how the lung allocates *qi*, those organs that need more get more and that need less get less. 'Fundamental Questions: Special Discussion on Meridians and Vessels' reads: 'The equilibrium of *qi* is reflected on the pulse at the *qi* opening (of the Lung Meridian of Hand Greater *Yin*). The pulse condition can determine a patient's death or survival.' The allocation of *qi* to all organs is regulated and orderly, so it is balanced. The pulse at the *qi* opening is what we call wrist pulse, the pulsation of the radial artery that can be felt at the wrist.

TCM doctors would feel the wrist pulse of a patient when making diagnoses. Some people consider it a magic or a wonder. Wrist pulse is on the lung meridian, so TCM doctors could get to know the lung condition of a patient by feeling this pulse. They could obtain a general understanding of the nutrition allocation in all organs. If those organs that need more get less, or those that need less get more, then diseases of the corresponding organs can occur. Therefore, various diseases can be diagnosed from wrist pulse. This is what was previously mentioned: the lung governs management and regulation. The lung regulates all organs in the human body to ensure them to work in a peaceful order. Then these organs will be able to fulfill their roles. This is the function of diffusion and dispersion.

The other aspect is that the lung governs depuration and descent. After diffusion and dispersion, *qi* goes downward, so this function is to descend *qi* movement. As the lyrics of a song[①] go, the cough disappears when *qi* moves smoothly from upward

---

① song: *Liquor Divine Melody* (酒神曲), a song of a 1987 Chinese movie *Red Sorghum* based on the novel *Red Sorghum Clan* by Nobel laureate Mo Yan (莫言).

to downward. The two aspects of the function that the lung governs, diffusion and dispersion as well as depuration and descent, should work in cooperation, and fulfill a complete *qi* activity involving both upward and downward movements. If problems occur in one aspect, the lung may have dysfunction. If the lung fails to depurate and descend, then tightness in the chest, difficulty breathing, reverse flow of *qi*, and coughing may occur. In severe cases, constipation can present.

According to *Huangdi's Inner Canon of Medicine*, *qi* movement of the *zang-fu* organs involves ascending, descending, exiting, and entering. The organs in the upper part need to descend *qi* and those in the lower part need to ascend *qi*. However, as far as an organ itself is concerned, it should involve both the ascent and the descent of *qi*. In other words, the dual flow of *qi* should be present in each organ. That is why the lung is said to govern diffusion and dispersion as well as depuration and descent. This is the dialectics expressed in *Huangdi's Inner Canon of Medicine*: not to see things in an absolute manner.

Q8. What does it mean that all meridians and vessels converge in the lung?

The lung acting as the prime minister assists the monarch (heart) in promoting blood circulation throughout the body. According to 'Fundamental Questions: Special Discussion on Meridians and Vessels,' 'all meridians and vessels converge in the lung (*fèi cháo bǎi mài* 肺朝百脉).' *Chao* (朝) generally means court meeting. In ancient China, all officials needed to attend the morning meeting to report to the emperor and receive instructions from the emperor. This meeting was organized by the prime minister. Hence it is believed that all meridians and vessels meet in the lung. The *qi* and blood in the entire body flow to the lung. Only when *qi* and blood reach the lung can the lung disperse turbid substances and *qi* out of the body and absorb fresh air from nature into the blood and then distribute it to the whole body. As a result, it is very important for all meridians and vessels to converge in the lung.

Some annotators think that *chao* not only means court meeting, but also refers to tidewater. That is, the lung could drive the *qi* and blood in all meridians and vessels to move in a regular pattern like tidewater. Some people call it 'lung *qi*' which serves as the dynamic force for *qi* and blood movement.

You may get confused at this point. It was mentioned in the previous chapters that the heart is the monarch, and it governs blood and vessels, which means the heart promotes the flow of *qi* and blood. But in this chapter about the physiological function of the lung, it is said that pectoral *qi* which consists of the inhaled fresh air and the *qi* derived from food and drinks promotes *qi* and blood movement. This begets the question: Does the heart promote the movement of *qi* and blood? The answer is yes. The heart indeed promotes *qi* and blood movement.

According to *Huangdi's Inner Canon of Medicine*, the heart is the monarch whose major responsibility is to govern spirit, including people's thought, mind, will, and thinking. Spirit, the intangible, is believed to control the body, the tangible; this is the key point. That what takes control is the monarch. As far as promoting *qi* and blood movement is concerned, it is routine work. The heart, being the monarch, should take responsibility, but the lung is the executive officer. Hence, the lung, being the prime minister, assists the heart in promoting the flow of *qi* and blood. If you happen to know a little about TCM, you might know that *Huangdi's Inner Canon of Medicine* proposes an ebb-flow doctrine of *qi* and blood in the twelve primary meridians, also known as the big cycle of the twelve meridians. The cycle begins with the Lung Meridian of Hand Greater *Yin*. Then *qi* and blood flow to the Large Intestine Meridian of Hand *Yang* Brightness, the Stomach Meridian of Foot *Yang* Brightness, the Spleen Meridian of Foot Greater *Yin*, the Heart Meridian of Hand Lesser *Yin*, the Small Intestine Meridian of Hand Greater *Yang*, the Bladder Meridian of Foot Lesser *Yang*, the Kidney Meridian of Foot Lesser *Yin*, the Pericardium Meridian of Hand Reverting *Yin*, the Triple Energizer Meridian of Hand Lesser *Yang*, the Gallbladder Meridian of Foot Lesser *Yang*, the Liver Meridian of Foot Reverting *Yin*, and back to the lung meridian, starting another cycle. The ebb and flow of *qi* and blood is in infinite cycle. This explains why it is said that the lung promotes *qi* and blood movement. (See Figure 13-1)

Another point is particularly interesting. You can feel the pounding of your heart below your left breast. As you may know, it is the pulsation at the apex of the heart. According to 'Fundamental Questions: Pulse Conditions of Healthy People,' 'the great collateral of the stomach is called *xu li* (虚里 , the area of the apex beat)...

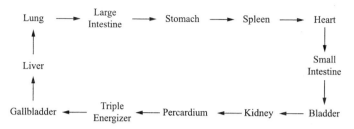

Figure 13-1   The ebb-flow of *qi* and blood in the twelve meridians

Its pulsation can reflect the condition of pectoral *qi*'. That is, feeling the apical pulse can help you differentiate between deficiency and excess of pectoral *qi*. As mentioned before, pectoral *qi* consists of the inhaled fresh air and the essential *qi* derived from food and drinks. It is formed in the chest and governed by the lung and the stomach. Pectoral *qi* permeates the heart and vessels to promote the flow of *qi* and blood.

Therefore, according to *Huangdi's Inner Canon of Medicine*, the promotion of *qi* and blood flow is accomplished by the heart with the help of the lung. It is for this reason that lung disorders can directly affect the flow of *qi* and blood and affect the heart. There is pulmonary heart disease in clinical practice. Lesions of the lung such as bronchitis and emphysema can affect the heart, leading to right ventricular hypertrophy and expansion, and finally causes right heart failure.

Some patients have a cough, dyspnea and feel lack of strength. They look very thin and weak, with a darkish complexion, blue lips, purple tongue, and sublingual veins as well as purple fingernails. They usually present the status of hypoxia, with poor blood circulation. The barrel chest indicates long-time emphysema. Due to persistent coughing and panting, the lung disease affects the heart at last, resulting in the disorder of *qi*-blood circulation. Therefore, the lung, regarded as the prime minister, exerts many effects on the heart, which should arouse our attention.

Q9. What does it mean that the lung governs regulation of water passage?

As is stated in 'Fundamental Questions: Special Discussion on Meridians and Vessels,' 'the lung regulates water passage and transports water to the bladder.' This is a major physiological function of the lung, which should be emphasized.

You may know that up to 70% of the human body is water. That is, you are made up mostly of fluids. Within these fluids, there is water besides blood. The regulation of water passage is accomplished by the lung, which is part of its job of assisting the heart.

In daily life, you will sweat in hot weather or after doing a large amount of exercise. In this situation, you may drink some water to maintain the balance of water metabolism in your body. Otherwise, you can also drink some hot tea or soup to sweat, which is also an important way to regulate the metabolism of your body fluids. The regulation is done not only through sweating, but also through urination and exhaling water vapor. Among them, sweating and urination are particularly involved in regulation.

Huangdi's Inner Canon of Medicine states that people sweat more in hot weather or when they wear more clothes; as a result, urine output is decreased. In cold weather or when people wear less clothes, people seldom sweat, and urine output is increased. In fact, sweat and urine can be transformed into each other. Some people think that the composition of sweat and that of urine are similar. So, if uremia patients can be treated with kidney dialysis, then they can be treated with skin dialysis, which is to make the patients sweat.

How can the water contained in food and drinks after ingestion be transformed into fluids and then regulated by the lung? In fact, when the food and drinks enter the stomach, the stomach would decompose them, and then the spleen transforms and transports the water fluids to the lung. The lung disperses them to the whole body for regulation. The *zang-fu* organs absorb the nutrients of water fluids. The remaining turbid *qi* and residues are removed out of the body either in the form of urine or sweat.

This process is explained in *Huangdi's Inner Canon of Medicine*. As 'Fundamental Questions: Special Discussion on Meridians and Vessels' states, 'when water is taken into the stomach, the essential *qi* is distributed and transported to the spleen. The spleen distributes the essence and transports it upwards to the lung. The lung regulates water passage and transports water downward to the urinary bladder. The essence of water is distributed all through the body and into the five meridians.'

To summarize, water is transformed into fluids and given to the lung by the spleen. The lung disperses them to the whole body and transports the waste to the bladder or transforms them into sweat to be removed out of body. This is the whole process of water metabolism, which has a close relationship with the lung.

In terms of water regulation, I would like to mention one more thing. Clinically, there are edema patients with an enlarged head and face and swollen eyes. When you press their shins for a few seconds, a pit will appear. They usually report that they have inhibited urination and their urine output is reduced. How do physicians treat these patients? According to 'Fundamental Questions: Soups and Liquors,' the therapeutic methods include 'opening sweat pores and cleaning the bladder.' The former is the method for inducing perspiration and the latter for promoting urination.

I'd like to dwell on the method of inducing perspiration. The purpose of this method is to ventilate the lung, to diffuse lung *qi* to sweat. It doesn't mean dispelling water through sweat pores. Since sweat is related to urine output, inducing sweating can contribute to the relief of inhibited urination. You may have experience in using a kettle or a teapot. As you know, there is a small hole in its lid. Without the hole, water cannot come out of a well-sealed kettle or teapot. This small hole is called air passage. TCM believes that the lung is in the upper energizer and is the canopy above, which is like the small hole in the lid of a kettle. If the lung is not opened, it means the hole is blocked and then the urination is impeded. Ancient Chinese people named it the method of lifting off the lid of a kettle. Urination is promoted through ventilating the lung, but not through increasing urination. This method can be used to treat edema. On one hand, through inducing perspiration, water fluids can be expelled; on the other hand, lung *qi* is diffused to expel the water through urination.

In the Qing dynasty, there was a famous TCM doctor named Zhang Zhicong (张志聪). He once treated a very typical edema patient who had had this disease for a long time. The patient received no effective treatment after visiting many well-known doctors, who used such formulas as Eight-ingredient Ratification Powder (*Bā Zhèng Săn* 八正散) to promote urination. The patient finally turned to Zhang Zhicong for help. Zhang decided to regulate the lung after diagnosis. He used the 'lifting-off-the-lid-of-a-kettle' method and prescribed three herbs of same dose to diffuse lung *qi*: Apricot Seed (*xìng rén* 杏仁), Divaricate Saposhnikovia Root, and

Perilla Leaf (*sū yè* 苏叶). After the patient took the medicine, urination was promoted and his edema was cured. Another formula named Maidservant from Yue Decoction (*Yuè Bì Tāng* 越婢汤), which is included in *Treatise on Cold Damage*, is also very effective in treating edema. It is used to diffuse lung *qi* and thus treat abnormal urination.

However, caution should be taken. Edema is a complicated disorder. If one has edema, they should visit doctors without delay and be diagnosed and treated based on pattern differentiation. Patients should not take medicines without seeking medical consultation.

Q10. How do you preserve lung health?

Here, I have to mention the air-quality issue. Recently, air pollution has become a hot topic. Fog is the result of water meeting cold air, which doesn't bring heavy pollution. Smog, a mix of smoke and fog, however, brings great harm to health. The main sources of smog include emission from chemical plants, vehicle exhaust, smoke from heating supply plants, and blowing dust. People would feel much more distressed when the smog becomes increasingly serious. When PM 2.5 rises to 100, you can see some office workers wear masks.

In fact, a lot of things in our daily life are no less harmful than smog, for instance, smoke from cigarettes and cooking oil. Speaking of tobacco smoke, if you smoke a cigarette in a house, the PM 2.5 can be off the charts. Statistics show that lighting a cigarette in a 35 m^2 room could increase the PM 2.5 level to four times greater than the normal safety level. Moreover, tobacco smoke is rich in many substances that harm the human body. The same is true of kitchen smoke. When delicious food is cooked, a lot of smoke can be produced, which rapidly increases PM 2.5, and it also contains many harmful substances.

Smog affects your body greatly. On one hand, the particulate matter enters your body and attaches to your respiratory tract. Some harmful substances can be absorbed. On the other hand, smog is also called brown cloud of the atmosphere. Smog weakens ultraviolet layer closer to the ground and reduces its sterilization effects. As a result, bacteria and pathogens will increase their activity. It will be easier for them to attach to particulate matters which will be absorbed by people. Hence, it is likely that more people contract infection. That is why you can see more patients with respiratory problems in the hospital when smog is heavy.

To protect your lungs, you should do the following things.

First, be a green commuter. You may drive private cars less frequently and take public transportation instead. If possible, walk.

Second, reduce tobacco smoke. Beijing has started implementing a smoking ban, so smokers must abide by this regulation and not smoke in indoor public places. Smoking is indeed a great harm to the human body.

Third, reduce cooking smoke. Discipline yourself. Adjust your eating habits. Try to reduce the intake of barbecued, grilled, or fried food.

Chapter 14
The Delicate Lung

Q1. What are the functions of the lung?

According to *Huangdi's Inner Canon of Medicine*, the five *zang*-organs make up a small empire, in which the lung is likened to the prime minister, who not only answers the call of the monarch—the heart, but also governs all the other organs of the body. TCM believes that the lung not only controls breathing and governs *qi*, but also propels the flow of *qi* and blood as well as regulates the waterways.

Q2. What is the lung's particular feature?

At the mention of the prime minister, you might think of the Chinese saying that 'a prime minister's mind is broad enough for poling a boat' which means magnanimousness. Nevertheless, TCM believes that the lung is delicate, apt to fall ill. There are two reasons for this. First, the lung lobes are delicate, susceptible to cold, heat, dryness, and dampness. Next, the lung is connected to the nose and governs skin and body hair, which are closely connected with nature, and thus vulnerable to various external pathogens. Therefore, the lung is also known as the delicate organ in TCM.

Q3. What does it mean that the lung governs skin and body hair?

As the idiom goes, 'a man knows by himself whether he feels cold or warm.' That is, the skin is the first sensor that allows you to feel heat, cold, tactile feedback, and pain. When you experience fear or fright, a cold gust of wind or an unexpected temperature drop, you often feel that a shiver comes over you before you get goose bumps. In fact, your muscles and skin shiver automatically to generate heat to maintain your body temperature. Likewise, in a hot environment, you sweat via the pores in your skin to keep your body temperature normal. That is why the skin is said to be the first line of contact with the external environment.

Huangdi's Inner Canon of Medicine believes that people may contract illnesses when pathogens such as wind, rain, cold, summer-heat, dryness, dampness and/ or fire invade the skin. According to 'Miraculous Pivot: The Occurrence of All Diseases' (*Líng Shū Bǎi Bìng Shǐ Shēng* 灵枢·百病始生), 'the invasion of deficiency-pathogen into the human body begins from the skin. When the skin is relaxed, the muscular interstice will be open. When it is open, pathogens will enter from body hair.' The expression 'deficiency-pathogen' refers to the pathogens in the external environment. When the sweat pores on the skin dilate, pathogens enter the human body through them and go all the way into its depths.

Such an important line of defense as the skin is under the charge of the lung. As 'Fundamental Questions: Flaccidity' reads, 'the lung governs skin and body hair.' Besides, 'Fundamental Questions: Various Relationships of the Five *Zang*-Organs' states: 'The lung is paired with skin, and it manifests its splendor on body hair.' To summarize, the lung is related to skin and body hair.

Q4. Why is it said that the lung governs skin and body hair?

There are two reasons. On the one hand, the lung governs diffusion and dispersion. It distributes the essence of food and drinks and inhaled clear *qi* to every part of the body including skin and body hair. In other words, skin and body hair depend on the lung for nourishment. Meanwhile, the lung also spreads defense *qi* to the surface of the human body and regulates the opening and closing of sweat pores.

On the other hand, the theory that the lung is closely related to skin and body hair is derived from daily experiences and observations. As is often observed, once people feel a chill and get goose bumps, they are prone to have a fever, a sore throat, or a cough later. That is the way external pathogens invade the body from the most external part—the skin to the lung, affecting its respiratory function, from which the ancient Chinese deduced the close connection between the lung and skin. Honestly, many TCM theories are summarized from observations and based on clinical experiences, making it a discipline of practice.

A common example of pathogens traveling from the skin to the lung is the common cold. Almost everyone has caught a cold at some point in their life. For instance, after rushing into heavy rain or a strong wind, people might find themselves coughing, running a fever, or feeling cold. That is how they catch a cold: they have exposure to external pathogens. Their symptoms can be diverse: nasal congestion, runny nose, itchy throat, cough, aversion to the cold and wind, and so on. With the passage of time, fever, severe coughing, and a sore throat may occur. TCM doctors believe that the disease is in the lung, skin as well as body hair though the pathogen makes its way through the skin.

Q5. Why do excellent doctors treat diseases when pathogenic factors have just invaded the skin and body hair?

'Fundamental Questions: Significant Discussions on Phenomena Corresponding to *Yin* and *Yang*' reads, 'expert doctors treat a disease when it is in the skin and body hair; next are those who treat a disease when it is in the muscles, then the doctors who treat a disease when it is in the sinews and meridians, then the doctors who treat a disease when it is in the six *fu*-organs, and finally the doctors who treat a disease when it is in the five *zang*-organs. Once the five *zang*-organs are involved, the chances of death and survival are half and half.' In other words, an excellent doctor, who excels at diagnosing and treating illnesses in their earliest phase, understands the urgency of taking measures when pathogens have just invaded the skin, to prevent them from going deeper. Again, we can conclude that skin is the first gate to shut external pathogens out.

Q6. What is the treatment strategy when pathogenic factors are in the skin?

According to 'Fundamental Questions: Significant Discussions on Phenomena Corresponding to *Yin* and *Yang*,' 'if the pathogenic factors are in the skin, sweating therapy can be used.' When the location of disease is relatively shallow, at the superficies, for instance, doctors should make the best use of the situation and make the patient sweat to expel the pathogens. Quite a few people have the habit of drinking a bowl of ginger decoction with brown sugar after catching a common cold due to their exposure to heavy rain or high winds. As *Huangdi's Inner Canon of Medicine* states, the pungent flavor governs dispersion. Fresh Ginger, pungent in flavor and warm in nature, facilitates sweating because of its dispersing effect. In addition, pungent medicinals enter the lung meridian, which enhances the diffusion and dispersion of lung *qi* to propel pathogens out.

It is worth mentioning that TCM and Western medicine adopt different ways of thinking in terms of relieving disorders. Rather than suppressing and eliminating the pathogens in the treatment, TCM targets their way out. On one hand, TCM doctors take measures to clear the passage for the exit of pathogens; on the other hand, they utilize medicinals to drive pathogens out from inside the body. Specifically, diaphoretic method, emesis or purgation can be used to expel the pathogens.

In 1950s, a Japanese Encephalitis (JE) epidemic occurred in China. With the failure of finding a cure in Western medicine, people resorted to a distinguished TCM physician, Pu Fuzhou (蒲辅周). An unexpectedly simple decoction he gave, the White Tiger Decoction, suppressed the JE epidemic like magic. It includes four ingredients: Gypsum, Common Anemarrhena Rhizome, Non-glutinous Rice (*jīng mǐ* 粳米), and Licorice Root, used to clear heat and generate fluids. People in the line of Western medicine were shocked at the result and they ran hundreds of tests to try to figure out how the White Tiger Decoction kills the JE virus. The conclusion is nevertheless the decoction does not function to kill the virus.

Perhaps an analogy can explain the difference between TCM and Western medicine in terms of treatment strategy. That is, contracting an illness is like growing crops. The virus or bacteria can be compared to plant seeds. There must be appropriate soil for the seeds to sprout, grow, and harvest. Likewise, pathogenic microorganisms require a suitable environment in the human body to develop. In the treatment, the seeds are what Western medicine is focused on, which need to be destroyed and killed. In contrast, the soil or the environment is what TCM targets and it believes that altering the growth environment can nip the seeds in the bud. That is the difference in the underlying philosophy of the two medical systems.

Q7. What is the well-known formula to treat people who are susceptible to catching a cold?

Some people are extremely intolerant of wind and coldness and may sweat even with light exertion. Others may sweat with no activity at all. Still others are susceptible to catching a cold and wouldn't recover until a couple of weeks or even months later. In TCM, this type of common cold is called 'the weak people's cold,' especially referring to those who have lung-*qi* deficiency. A formula is specially dedicated to this case, that is, Jade Wind-Barrier Powder (*Yù Píng Fēng Săn* 玉屏风散), which is used to replenish *qi*, consolidate the superficies, and arrest perspiration.

The Jade Wind-Barrier Powder is made up of Milkvetch Root, White Atractylodes Rhizome, Divaricate Saposhnikovia Root, and Fresh Ginger. As the lung governs the pectoral *qi* that consists of not only the clear *qi* from respiration but also the nutrients from food and drinks, the tonification of spleen *qi* is indispensable. Thus, while Milkvetch Root nurtures lung *qi*, White Atractylodes Rhizome functions as the tonic of spleen *qi*. And there is Divaricate Saposhnikovia Root. With a dispersing effect of expelling the pathogens, it brings the strengthened *qi* to consolidate the exterior. Fresh Ginger is another ingredient with a dispersing effect. The four ingredients work together to tonify lung *qi*, disperse *qi* to the skin and body hair to strengthen their defense and expel possible pathogens. It is very effective to cure weak people with a cold. Just like how a wind-barrier shields the wind, it defends the human body against external pathogens.

By the way, I would like to bring your attention to one thing. Some people hastily take off their coats after intense activity. For example, some children like to take off their coat after playing games, and even rush to an air-conditioned room to cool down. This is utterly inadvisable. Due to the dilation of sweat pores after all those activities and sweating, environmental pathogens would easily break through the barrier of human skin, slip through the pores, and invade the body. In this case, common cold may occur.

Q8. What is the relationship between the lung and the large intestine?

Apart from performing its normal defensive function, healthy skin is one of the major factors that contribute to one's beauty. Possessing a good look is one thing. Only when it is combined with perfect glowing skin can the look really be flattered, presenting a heavenly sight.

Then, what affects the skin?

One factor is defecation. People with rough skin, pigmentation, spots, or facial acne are often pestered by constipation or difficulty in defecation. It is universally known that one cannot live without air or food. The clear *qi* is inhaled, while the turbid *qi* is breathed out. If the turbid *qi* fails to leave the body, it will become waste products and turn into toxins. The same is true with food and drinks. As their nutrients are assimilated, the remaining waste is to be eliminated from the body. In the body, the lung is responsible for expelling the waste air, whilst the large intestine takes charge of removing food residues. In *Huangdi's Inner Canon of Medicine*, there is a well-known theory—'the lung is interior-exteriorly related to the large intestine.' Why is it?

The lung is located in the upper part of the body, and the large intestine is in the lower part. How come they are interior-exteriorly related? *Huangdi's Inner Canon of Medicine* believes in the pairing of *zang*-organs and *fu*-organs. According to

'Miraculous Pivot: Meridians,' 'the Lung Meridian of Hand Greater *Yin* originates from the middle energizer, running downward to connect with the large intestine. Winding back, it goes along the upper orifice of the stomach, passes through the diaphragm, and enters the lung.' That is to say, the lung and the large intestine are directly linked by the meridian, thus they are interior-exteriorly related.

Another perspective that explains the relationship between the lung and the large intestine lies in the lung's functions. As the lung governs diffusion and dispersion, it spreads the nutrients and body fluids to every part of the human body, down to the bowels. Besides, the lung also governs depuration and descent, so it facilitates the large intestine's downward movement to improve defecation.

The last and the most important reason, like most TCM theories, is based on clinical experiences. It was often observed by the ancient Chinese that patients with lung heat, manifesting typical symptoms such as a flushed face, hot, rapid and smelly breath, sore throat, and coughs, had trouble defecating. Problems related to the lung won't be resolved completely until bowel movement returns to normal. Hence, the ancients deduced the interior-exterior relationship between the lung and the large intestine. Accordingly, if you want to have healthy skin, you should not only have the lung nourished, but keep your bowel movements normal.

Over a decade ago there was a popular capsule in China called the Detox and Beauty Capsule (*Pái Dú Yǎng Yán Jiāo Náng* 排毒养颜胶囊)[1], which was derived from a formula designed by Prof. Jiang Liangduo (姜良铎) at the First Affiliated Hospital of Beijing University of Chinese Medicine. As the name suggests, beauty can be obtained through detoxification. By restoring normal function of the large intestine, your skin will glow naturally—that is the rationale behind it.

Above are the three reasons why the lung is closely related to the large intestine.

---

① Detox and Beauty Capsule (*Pái Dú Yǎng Yán Jiāo Náng* 排毒养颜胶囊) contains Rhubarb and is a heat-clearing and laxative herbal medicine. People are advised to consult a TCM practitioner before taking it.

Q9. What does it mean that the lung opens into the nose?

The bond between the nose and the lung is inseparable. According to 'Miraculous Pivot: Length of Meridians,' 'lung *qi* communicates with the nose and only when the lung is in harmony can the nose distinguish odor from aroma.' Being the supplier and the governor of the nose, the lung transports clear *qi* to the nose to permit normal olfactory function. In turn, the nose reciprocates by altering the humidity and temperature of the air traveling in the nasal cavity. Dirty particles are filtered by cilia and adhered to the secreted mucus to protect the lung from potential harm. Otherwise, external pathogens may enter from the nose to invade the lung and cause illnesses. For instance, it is very likely that droplet infections cause some lung disorders.

When there are nasal disorders such as nasal obstruction, a runny nose, nasal dryness, or impaired sense of smell, physicians can target at the lung in treatment. A runny nose, for instance, is common at the onset of a cold. The patient may experience nasal obstruction at first, then have a runny nose with clear nasal discharge, and then have yellowish turbid nasal discharge after a few more days. With the method of diffusing the lung, some patients might have their colds cured, and those nasal symptoms might disappear. However, for some other people, nasal problems such as profuse nasal discharge may remain and linger until escalating into rhinitis.

A couple of months ago, a friend of mine took his child to my consultation room for treatment. The child sneezed every morning after getting up. Every time he had to sneeze for seven to ten times, and then kept having a runny nose with clear nasal discharge. The condition had persisted for as long as half a year. Moreover, due to his itchy nose, the child developed a habit of rubbing his nose and eyes until they turned red. Medicine for a cold was taken but no good results were obtained. Later, he developed night cough and wheezing that lasted for a while. He was then suspected of having bronchitis and thus was given infusion and antibiotics, but none of the methods worked. Finally, he was brought to visit me. The child was diagnosed with allergic rhinitis. According to TCM theory that the lung controls the nose, the child in fact had deficiency of lung *qi*. When lung *qi* is not consolidated, problems in the nasal cavity can occur. For this child, I prescribed the Jade Wind-Barrier Powder with the addition or subtraction of some medicinals.

In ancient times, there was a famous medical book entitled *Classified Medical Records of Distinguished Physicians* (*Míng Yī Lèi Àn* 名医类案) in which a similar case was documented. A patient had a runny nose for three years and no cure was obtained. Later, he went to visit a well-known physician, who gave him a prescription with the following four ingredients: Biond Magnolia Flower (*xīn yí* 辛夷), Siberian Cocklebur Fruit (*cāng ěr zǐ* 苍耳子), Peppermint, and Dahurian Angelica Root (*bái zhǐ* 白芷). After some time, the symptom gradually disappeared, and so did his nasal itch. All the ingredients enter the lung meridian, working on the diffusion and dispersion of lung *qi* and promoting lung *qi* to reach the nasal cavity for a successful cure.

If you have allergic rhinitis, you ought to seek medical consultation instead of blindly copying the aforementioned prescription, because TCM believes that treatment should be given only after pattern differentiation is made and every prescription ought to be individualized. For example, those with a bright pale complexion and intolerance of cold may be deficient in *yang*, and are to be cured by supplementing *yang* to boost immunity rather than nourishing the lung.

In terms of sneezing, it is more than just a symptom in TCM. Sneezing is an alarming signal of the invasion of pathogens. Also, according to 'Miraculous Pivot: Questions and Answers,' 'the smooth flow of *yang qi* distributes all over the chest and rushes out of the nose and causes sneezing.' If *yang qi* flows smoothly, it functions normally in expelling the internal pathogens and sneezing is the manifestation that is observed.

Accordingly, sneezing is regarded as a good sign at the onset of a cold, which means healthy *qi* is doing its part of expelling pathogens. Upon sneezing, you need to bring your attention to it. It is best to keep the body warm or take some medications to prevent further development of the discomfort.

Q10. What does it mean that the lung governs the autumn season?

Autumn spans the seventh, the eighth, and the ninth months in lunar calendar. As the autumn wind blows, summer-heat and dampness get swept away, bringing cool weather with less humidity. According to TCM theory, autumn is the season when *yin qi* grows and *yang qi* declines. You can see the drooping and falling of leaves and branches. As for the human body, dryness-related symptoms can occur such as itchy and dry throat and skin, dry tongue and mouth, and increased difficulty in defecation.

All these dryness symptoms, according to TCM theory, are related to the lung. So, what do you do about it, to prevent and cure it? Some experienced people would suggest replenishing the fluids to combat dryness. Drinking more water will help, and so will eating more juicy pears. Some medicinals such as Dwarf Lilyturf Root, Asparagus Root (*tiān dōng* 天冬), and Adenophora Root (*shā shēn* 沙参) can be added to soup to help increase body fluids. The above methods do affect some people, while other individuals may see no effect at all. Why is that?

Huangdi's Inner Canon of Medicine provides another way to interpret dryness and the dominant *qi* of autumn. It believes that autumn corresponds to the lung, which pertains to the element of metal. Metal or lung *qi* is characterized by descension. Also, TCM believes that the left ascends, and the right descends. As the lung is stored on the right, lung *qi* is expected to flow downward. If so, can fluids be efficiently diffused and dispersed?

A phenomenon may help to illustrate this theory. If you wish to bring a tree with drooping leaves and fallen branches back to life, can you achieve that by simply watering it? Will its leaves turn green and branches grow? Negative. It is not the lack of water that takes the vitality away; rather, the inefficiency of obtaining nourishments is the root cause. Accordingly, to relieve dryness in the human body, lung *qi* must be dispersed to nourish its related body parts. Medicinals such as Perilla Leaf, Platycodon Root (*jié gěng* 桔梗), Hogfennel Root (*qián hú* 前胡), and Apricot Seed are frequently used to diffuse lung *qi*, facilitating better dispersion of fluids in the human body so that dryness can be alleviated.

Q11. What do you do to nurture the lung in autumn?

A well-quoted saying can be found in 'Fundamental Questions: Significant Discussions on Regulating the Spirit in Accordance with the *Qi* of the Four Seasons.' 'The three months of autumn are the season of harvest. The *qi* of heaven becomes tense, and the *qi* of the earth is clear. People should sleep early at night and rise early in the morning like roosters. They should keep their mind at peace to alleviate the binding effect of cool autumn *qi*, gather their spirit and *qi* to make autumn *qi* balanced, and prevent outward manifestation of their sentiments to make lung *qi* clear. This is the way to adapt to autumn *qi* and preserve gathering.'

The above quote makes clear the following points.

First, when *yang qi* declines and *yin qi* increases in autumn, activities should be reduced and time for rest should be increased.

Second, phrased as 'rise early in the morning like roosters,' what it attempts to convey is that people should follow the laws of nature. According to the ancient Chinese, animals surpass human beings in following natural rules and principles. Humans, however, are too complicated and strong-minded to follow nature. Therefore, compliance with nature is what you should try to work towards.

Third, in terms of mindset and mood, you should keep your mind at peace, gather your spirit and *qi*, and do not expose your desires or intentions. As far as ideas or intentions are concerned, they are generated in spring, exhibited in summer, restrained in autumn, and concealed in winter. So, in autumn, do not give in to your desires.

As was mentioned at the beginning of this chapter, the lung plays a vital role in the body system. It is compared to the prime minister in an empire of the human body, who not only answers the call of the monarch—the heart, but also governs all the other officials or multiple organs of the body. Governing the first line of defense—the skin and connected to the nose, the lung is susceptible to diseases. Hence, you have to observe the following three points to take good care of the lung.

To begin with, do exercises to improve lung function. You can climb hills, swim, go biking, play ball and so on. Doing sports can help you increase your vital capacity and strengthen lung function so that you'll be better able to guard against external pathogens. Among various sports, swimming is highly recommended, which is the best way to increase lung capacity.

Next, contribute to the improvement of air quality. As the lungs control breathing and have direct communication with the air, the impact of air quality on the lungs is unparalleled. In a broader sense, people should combat heavy smog as soon as possible. For every individual, there are things that can be improved in everyday life. For example, you can reduce the consumption of cigarettes, barbecues, and fried dishes. The better the air quality is, the healthier the lungs are.

Finally, ensure appropriate cold and heat stimulations. The lung governs the skin which is the first line of defense from external pathogens. The skin is highly sensitive to changes of temperature. By means of thermal stimulation, the adaptability and resilience of the skin will be amplified. That is why there will be a cold-water pool next to hot springs in some places, which allows you to experience cold water after plunging into hot water for adjustment and stimulation. This hot-to-cold experience is believed to be beneficial to your body.

In conclusion, you can strengthen your lung capacity and fortify the first line of defense through regular exercise and sufficient rest so that you can avoid pathogenic attacks and keep your lungs healthy.

Chapter 15

The Root of Prenatal Constitution: The Kidney

Q1. What is the kidney in TCM?

The concept of the kidney in TCM differs from that of Western medicine, which can be quite confusing. Many patients, upon hearing the TCM physician's diagnosis 'kidney deficiency,' would feel scared, fearing that their life is at stake since this vital organ has a problem. In Western medicine, kidneys refer to the two bean-shaped organs on the left and right sides of the body. They filter blood, maintain liquid equilibrium and electrolyte balance, have endocrine functions, and regulate blood pressure. The concept of the kidney in TCM, however, differs. It is rather invisible and intangible, referring to no specific organ. It is in fact a combination of multiple systems, including the nervous system, the immune system, the endocrine system and so on. Part of the combined function of the aforementioned systems is what we call the kidney in TCM. Unfortunately, TV advertisements of food supplements with kidney-nourishing effects often demonstrate a concrete image of the two kidneys, causing further misunderstanding amongst non-professionals. In Western medicine, indeed, kidney diseases often cannot be easily cured, demanding a myriad of medical tests and treatments. Kidney deficiency in TCM, however, can be cured with certain herbal medicines.

Q2. Why is the kidney termed the root of prenatal constitution?

In TCM, the kidney is termed '*xian tian zhi ben*' (先天之本, the root of prenatal constitution), which underscores its importance. 'Prenatal' means something that is already there before one's birth, without the interference of the environment afterwards. TCM believes that one's growth, physical appearance, and constitution all have to do with the kidney.

Why is the kidney referred to as the root of prenatal constitution? The answer lies in ancient Chinese culture. 'The Book of History: Great Principles' lists the sequence of the five elements as follows: 'The first is water, the second fire, the third wood, the fourth metal, and the fifth earth,' placing the element of water in the first place. Likewise, in the Chapter 'Water and Earth' (*Shuǐ Dì Piān*, 水地篇) in *Guanzi*, water is described as 'the root of all things,' occupying a central role. Of course, 'water' in ancient Chinese philosophy should be understood not simply as tangible water, but rather substances that share similar qualities with it. These substances are the origin of all living things. Human beings are part of the myriad beings, so they are no exception. That is, water is also the origin of humans. Since the ancient Chinese believed that the kidney governs water, it is therefore called the root of prenatal constitution. The spleen is referred to as 'the root of acquired constitution,' as has been elaborated on in previous chapters. As their terms suggest, the kidney and the spleen are dominant in health. However, their functions vary. The kidney determines one's life in the way that water gives life to all living things. The spleen, by comparison, nourishes the human body and maintains one's physical well-being in the way that earth nourishes myriad things.

Q3. What are the major functions of the kidney?

In this chapter, two of the kidney's major functions are discussed. First, the kidney has an impact on inheritance. Second, the kidney plays a significant role in one's life from birth, to growth, maturity, senility, and finally death.

Q4. How does the kidney impact inheritance?

According to 'Miraculous Pivot: Natural Span of Life,' Huangdi asked Qibo: 'When life begins at conception, what *qi* is the foundation? What *qi* is the defense?' Qibo answered: 'The mother's *qi* constitutes the foundation; the father's *qi* serves as defense.' Therefore, the ancient Chinese believed that a human embryo is formed by the mother's blood (*yin*) and the father's essence (*yang*). The merging of a mother and father's essential *qi* forms an embryo, which is called prenatal essence in TCM. Prenatal essence, originating from the reproductive essence, is stored in the kidney upon birth. Nowadays, people talk about information transmission. The kidney is in fact a medium of information transmission so that a child gets to inherit his parents' looks, regarded as the 'flesh and blood' of his parents. This is the ancients' way of explaining how the parents' genetic legacy is preserved and passed on to the next generation. Like DNA in modern science, prenatal essence in TCM theory has a huge impact on health, especially on the life span of a person.

The research conducted by the Soviet Union on the life expectancy of people in 5,000 families revealed that family members of those in the age bracket of 80 to 84 are 51% likely to be long-lived, and the longevity rate increases to over 70% for the families of those aged 105 and over. Genetic researchers had a follow-up study of 1,600 twins and found that the life span of identical twins was very close, with an average difference of merely 3 years for identical twins and 6 years for fraternal twins while that of siblings rises to 9 years. Therefore, genetics are a decisive factor in one's life span. Likewise, *Huangdi's Inner Canon of Medicine* attaches utmost importance to the kidney when it comes to preserving health, fending off diseases, and pursuing longevity.

Q5. What is the role of the kidney in one's different stages of life?

TCM believes that the kidney plays a significant role in one's growth, development, and reproduction. According to *Huangdi's Inner Canon of Medicine*, one's life span can be divided into several stages, each spanning ten years. This theory is based on years of observation and life experience. The kidney is thought to play a significant role in every stage. 'Miraculous Pivot: Natural Span of Life' reads: 'At the age of ten years old, one's five *zang*-organs have developed and are permeated with blood and *qi*. With the *qi* in the lower part, one tends to run.' During the time from one's birth to ten years old, one's five *zang*-organs begin to develop; *qi* and blood are on the increase. One's body, nevertheless, has not yet reached maturity. Kidney *qi* is mainly in the lower energizer; hence the child is inclined to run. This links kids' vivacity to their growing kidney *qi*.

The ancient Chinese referred to children as 'little *yin* and little *yang*' or immature *yin* and *yang*, meaning they haven't fully developed. Children's diseases are usually of simpler causes, conforming to the simple nature of childhood. Accordingly, herbal medicines for children tend to be light and simple, containing fewer herbs. It is rare for a TCM physician to prescribe a child medicinals for treatment that lasts more than two weeks. Often, a child falls ill due to either food retention in his stomach or catching a cold. Some Chinese grandparents tend to spoil their grandkids, constantly worrying that the children are hungry, feeding them with too much food. Once there is a slight change in weather, they would wrap the kids in many layers, which is highly unnecessary. Consequently, children are likely to suffer from the 'cold enveloping fire' syndrome. Those causes are not complicated, so children will restore health after being given such simple treatments as expelling retained food, reducing inner heat, and dissipating coldness.

Because the *qi*, blood, and *zang-fu* organs of a child have not reached maturity, his state of mind and mental activity are not complete either. Children are worry free. A simple comparison between primary school and college students would suffice as the obvious difference between a child and an adult. When the final class of a primary school day ends, pupils all run out with a great racket. In contrast, a university campus rarely witnesses such scenes. If a kid walks slowly with his head drooping and hands clasped behind his back, passers-by will wonder whether he/she is in trouble, because a normal kid never behaves like that. Children think and act like children. A schoolchild would rather first go out to play for a while and then come home to finish his homework, while his parents would prefer that he should do the reverse. Another example is the class length. Kindergarten classes last from twenty to thirty minutes per session, while in university that will double. In a word, kids by nature can hardly sit still.

Things are different in the following stages of life.

'Miraculous Pivot: Natural Span of Life' states that when one reaches 20, 'blood and *qi* begin to be abundant; flesh and muscles get stronger. Hence, one tends to walk briskly.' At the age of 30, 'the five *zang*-organs have reached maturity; muscles are strong; blood vessels are full and vigorous. Hence, one tends to walk.' That means people in their twenties or thirties are physically strong and they are vigorous in physical activities. Since they have a strong and healthy body, they rarely suffer from deficiency patterns. Most of their disorders fall into the category of excess patterns, and thus they do not need any tonifying therapy. However, youngsters' mental strength is yet to reach its peak, hence often in need of further instruction and experience.

The age of 40 is a milestone. 'Miraculous Pivot: Natural Span of Life' states that when one reaches 40, 'five *zang*-organs and six *fu*-organs as well as twelve meridians are at their peak and equally stable; muscular interstice begins to become flabby; skin loses its luster and vitality wanes; white hair starts to show; a normal abundance is reached, and no swaying exists. Hence, one tends to sit down.' At the age of 40, along with the exuberance of one's blood and *qi*, one's state of mind also reaches a sound stage. Therefore, one behaves prudently and tends to sit down. As Confucius said: 'At the age of 40, one has no doubts or misgivings.'

Nevertheless, decline begins when something reaches its peak. Although one is in his prime at the age of 40, aging starts to take its toll. This embodies the dialectical thoughts of TCM. As is stated in 'Fundamental Questions: Significant Discussions on Phenomena Corresponding to *Yin* and *Yang*,' for some people 'at the age of forty, half of *yin qi* has already been consumed; early aging begins to appear in one's daily activities.' In this quote, *yin qi* refers to kidney *qi* as the kidney pertains to *yin*. Along with the decline of kidney *qi*, the human body starts to decline in multiple ways. This explains why people after 40 years old seem to care and know more about health preservation. This age group is easily inclined to patronize the foot massage clinics that have mushroomed in China because they sense that there are certain age-related declines in some physiological functions. However, at this stage of life, it is better for one to seek regulation rather than use tonics.

After kidney *qi* starts to decline, which organ's *qi* declines next? The kidney pertains to water, and water generates wood. According to the five-element theory, the liver pertains to wood. So, in the following stage of life, when one reaches the age of 50, one's liver *qi* starts to decline. Wood generates fire, which is the heart, so at the age of 60, one's heart *qi* becomes insufficient. Fire generates earth, which is the spleen. Earth generates metal, which is the lung. When the circle is complete and comes back to water, that is, the kidney, one's life may come to an end.

'Miraculous Pivot: Natural Span of Life' states: 'When one is 50 years old, liver *qi* begins to decline, liver lobes become thinner, bile begins to decrease, and vision begins to blur.' At the age of 50, a common manifestation of the declining liver is one's eyesight begins to fade, as the liver governs eyes. It also governs tendons, so a person of 50 years old is not as physically flexible as before. A young adult may recover from a day's hard work with a good night's sleep, but this is no longer the case when one is in his forties or fifties.

At the age of 60, 'heart *qi* begins to decline; sadness and bitterness set in; blood and *qi* slow down. Hence, one tends to lie down.' The heart governs one's mental activity, so people in this stage are prone to depression and sentimentality, losing interest in past hobbies and preferring solitude. The heart also governs blood, so when one's blood flow is no longer smooth and easy, one does not feel like moving about.

At the age of 70, the text reads: 'spleen *qi* is deficient; the skin is withered.' The spleen governs flesh and muscles. If spleen *qi* is insufficient, a septuagenarian becomes flabby or sinewless.

At the age of 80, 'lung *qi* declines; corporeal soul departs. Hence one makes frequent mistakes when talking.' A significant function of the lung is that it houses the corporeal soul, which is 'what enters and leaves together with the combined essence,' as is said in 'Miraculous Pivot: Basic State of Spirit.' The combined essence refers to the embryo. When the fetus is developed, the functions of motor and sensory nerves present themselves. So, the corporeal soul is in the realm of spirit, referring to certain intuitive senses that one is born with, for instance, sensory perception and kinetic sense. Therefore, an octogenarian may experience the decline of such intuitions when lung *qi* declines. Alzheimer's disease is a case in point. News reports from previous years used to publicize the following story: An old man fell down on the street. When a passer-by helped him get back on his feet, he declared in the first place that the kindhearted stranger was the one that knocked him down. Some commentators categorized this behavior into moral degradation. In fact, sometimes, the senior citizen does not harbor any scheme in advance. Instead, he has a moment of his 'corporeal soul leaving the body,' like senile dementia. He may not know what he used to know and may not understand what he used to understand. In clinical practice, some of the patients at this stage of life will be diagnosed with dementia, with both his state of mind and behavior deviated from healthy ones. So, *Huangdi's Inner Canon of Medicine* describes people in their eighties as making 'frequent mistakes when talking.'

After a full cycle from the kidney to the liver, the heart, the spleen, and the lung, it comes back to the kidney. In the next stage of life, when one is in his nineties, he is very likely to suffer from greater deficiency in the kidney. As the text reads, 'at the age of 90, kidney *qi* is depleted, and the meridians of the other four *zang*-organs are empty and weak.' The kidney plays a pivotal role in one's growth and development. If kidney *qi* is exhausted, even if one still hangs on to life, it does not last long. 'At the age of 100, all five *zang*-organs are deficient; spirit *qi* disappears, leaving behind only the shell of a body. The life ends.' The physical body is the basis of the spirit. When the former is extremely weak and dying, so is the latter. That is, when all is gone, death ensues.

The life process from cradle to grave is reflected in a present-day jingle:

At birth, time for getting on the stage.

At ten, time for progressing every day.

At twenty, time for projecting lofty ideals.

At thirty, time for striving for success.

At forty, time for being popular and at ease.

At fifty, time for getting settled and peace.

At sixty, time for returning to private life.

At seventy, time for playing mahjong games.

At eighty, time for soaking up some sunshine.

At ninety, time for lying on one's bed.

At a hundred, time for departing the world.

Huangdi's Inner Canon of Medicine summarizes the human life from birth to death in 'Miraculous Pivot: Natural Span of Life' with 219 Chinese characters, giving great importance to the kidney, especially when the health is in decline from 40 years old onwards. The declining phase is the ongoing process of organs becoming deficient. As is stated in 'Fundamental Questions: Significant Discussions on Phenomena Corresponding to *Yin* and *Yang*,' it is termed 'deficiency in the lower part of the body and excess in the upper.' 'Deficiency in the lower part of the body' refers to the deficiency in the lower energizer, mainly kidney-*yang* deficiency, which will incur its inability to transform *yin*, and which takes shape in tangible matter, like nasal mucus, dribbling saliva, and profuse phlegm. These are the manifestations of the 'excess in the upper part of the body,' which are often seen in the elderly people. So, for those elder patients, physicians usually try to tonify their lower energizer with herbs warm in property.

Q6. What is the relationship between the kidney and reproduction?

The kidney is also known for its impact on reproduction. One paragraph in 'Fundamental Questions: Genuine *Qi* Endowed by Heaven in Remote Antiquity' is specially devoted to the elaboration on this issue. To mark milestones in the reproductive aspect, it divides a female's life into several phases on a seven-year basis, and a male's life on an eight-year basis. Hence there is the saying 'seven for female and eight for male.'

The text reads: 'In a female, at the age of seven, her kidney *qi* becomes prosperous; her teeth begin to change; her hair grows long. At the age of 14, *tian gui* matures; conception vessel is passable; thoroughfare vessel is vigorous; period occurs in due time. Hence, she can conceive a child.' The expression *tian gui* means heaven water, which is stored in the kidney. It promotes the reproductive function. When *tian gui*, the sex-stimulating substance, is mature, so is a female's reproductive function.

By the time three times seven[①] (21 years old) and four times seven (28 years old), kidney *qi* is in its prime. Both mark the vigorous and thriving phases of a woman's life. These are the best time for childbearing.

By the time five times seven (35 years old), '*yang* brightness meridian starts to decline; the face looks haggard.' It signals the decline of her reproductive function.

If a woman looks wan and sallow at the age of 35, then from five times seven (35 years old), to six times seven (42 years old), to seven times seven (49 years old), *tian gui*, the substance that promotes human reproductive function and that is closely related to kidney essence, is gradually in decline until it becomes exhausted. At that time, the text reads: 'The way of the earth is impassable, then a woman cannot conceive.' 'The way of the earth being impassable' refers to menopause. Therefore, her fertility is lost.

To sum up, for a female, the phase from one times seven, to two times seven, three times seven, four times seven, five times seven, six times seven, and finally to seven times seven marks the growth, abundance, reduction, decline, and cessation of her reproductive function.

For a male, the process of reproductive function from growth to maturity and then to decline is almost the same as that of a female, with the only difference of using eight instead of seven years as markers for division. During the first and the second eight years of a male's life, he will be growing. When he is 16 years old, kidney *qi* reaches its normal level and begins to be abundant. So, a man can produce children. The text reads: 'If he copulates with a woman in this period, he can have children.' During the third and the fourth eight years he will be in the prime of his life and his health will reach the summit in the fifth eight years when he is around

---

① seven: referring to seven years of age.

40 years old. During the sixth and the seventh eight years, his kidney *qi* will be in decline, and his reproductive function ends in the eighth eight years when he is about 64 years old.

The expression 'kidney *qi*' occurs frequently in this part of the text, for it is kidney *qi* that impacts the development and the changes of the reproductive system of human beings. When kidney *qi* is abundant, human reproductive function works well. When kidney *qi* declines, human reproductive function declines. When kidney *qi* is exhausted, human reproductive function stops working.

Q7. Why is there the saying 'seven for female and eight for male'?

Why did the ancient Chinese divide a female's life into several phases on a seven-year basis and the male's life on an eight-year basis? The primary contributor is what they had gathered from observation. Besides, it can be interpreted from the perspective of TCM. According to *Huangdi's Inner Canon of Medicine*, a female's body is thought to be 'the body of lesser *yin*' and a male's to be 'the body of lesser *yang*.' To trigger change in *yin*, *yang* is required. An odd number pertains to *yang*, that is why every seven (odd-numbered) years, major changes occur in a female's body. An even number pertains to *yin*, hence eight for male.

Q8. What can further be elaborated on kidney issues?

First, since the kidney plays a vital role in the change of reproductive function, the ancient Chinese took it very seriously to protect and preserve kidney *qi*. Tonifying the kidney may help improve reproductive function and delay its decline.

Second, the prime of one's reproductive function is between the ages from 21 to 28 for a woman, and 24 to 32 for a man. The recommended age group for a woman to conceive a baby is before the age of 35, and for a man before the age of 40, when kidney *qi* is relatively vigorous. After a woman is 35 years old or after a man is 40 years old, her or his kidney *qi* is in decline, and it may not be the best time to have a child anymore.

Third, climacterium is another thing worth mentioning. Menopause coincides with the 'seventh seven' when a woman is around 49 years old. For a man around 64, he is no longer vigorous in his reproductive function. This phase also sees changes in internal secretions, resulting in a change of temperament. So, people at this stage of life need to regulate their mood to better adapt to the physical changes.

Fourth, quite a few things are closely related to the kidney, for example, periods, teeth, and hair. Clinically, regulating the kidney is the guiding principle for treating symptoms including irregular menstruation and hair and teeth problems.

In fact, all the other organs, blood, and *qi*, are also closely related to the kidney. 'Fundamental Questions: Genuine *Qi* Endowed by Heaven in Remote Antiquity' states: 'The kidney controls water. It receives and stores essence from the five *zang*-organs and the six *fu*-organs. Thus, only when the five *zang*-organs and the six *fu*-organs are vigorous can the kidney have enough essence to discharge.' That is, the kidney (the root of prenatal foundation) is the basis for other *zang-fu* organs. Owing to this close connection, the kidney can be nurtured through the nurturing of other organs. There is a dialectical relationship between them. Above all, one can never emphasize too much the protection and the nurturing of the kidney, for it is the innate foundation, and of vital importance to health.

Chapter 16
The Kidney's Miraculous Effects

Q1. What does it mean that the lower back is the house of the kidney?

Kidney, the root of prenatal constitution, not only controls inheritance and reproduction, but also plays a decisive role in one's overall health. Moreover, its role as the water organ makes it more special, affecting quite several other aspects of human health.

Let's begin with the relationship between the kidney and the lower back. The kidney is in the lower back, according to the ancient Chinese. They believed that inflexibility of the lower back indicated kidney problems. 'Fundamental Questions: Essentials of Pulse Taking and the Subtleties of Pulse Manifestation' (*Sù Wèn Mài Yào Jīng Wēi Lùn* 素问•脉要精微论) states: 'The lower back is the house of the kidney. Inability to turn one's lower back indicates the kidney is in decline.' This opinion is backed by many examples. For instance, many senior citizens complain about soreness or pain in the lower back. Likewise, TCM physicians are no strangers to those patients who claim they have experienced soreness and weakness in the lower back and knees. Often, TCM physicians would attribute such symptoms in the lower back to kidney problems.

There was a seemingly bizarre case that may serve as proof. One winter, a young man experienced sudden lower back pain after having sex with his girlfriend. They were not married at the time, and the young man was scared for having premarital sex. At first, his pain could be relieved by slightly stooping his lower back, but then his condition deteriorated to such an extent that he could only bear it when bending all the way down. By the time he went to a clinic, he was bent over 150 degrees and walked into the consultation room with the support of others. Two factors brought on his condition. First, the fear for having premarital sex impaired his kidney, as TCM physicians believe that fear can impair the kidney function. The second reason has to do with the time of the year, winter, which features cold weather. In coldness, the collaterals and the meridians contracted, so the flow of *qi* and blood was impeded, impairing his kidney *qi*. That is why his lower back could not maintain flexibility and he had to stoop down. Once the mechanism of his condition was clear, he was treated by warming the kidney, promoting the flow of *yang qi* and blood circulation, and dissipating cold. After two weeks of treatment, the patient could stand up straight again. The treatment was effective since there was no damage in his lumbar vertebrae.

Of course, not all diseases in the lower back point to kidney problems. Also, it must be reiterated that the concept of the kidney in TCM differs from that in Western medicine. One cannot declare that lower back pains caused by such diseases as kidney stone or ureteral calculus are all manifestations of kidney deficiency. Usually, kidney deficiency-related lower back pain may be involved in some of the following diseases: nephritis, certain gynecological diseases, strain of lumbar muscles, prostatitis and so on. One must always remember that when someone is diagnosed by a TCM physician to have kidney deficiency, it does not necessarily mean that he or she needs to have renal function tests and receive treatment for the actual organ.

Q2. How does kidney *qi* impact hearing ability?

In TCM, ears are governed by the kidney. 'Miraculous Pivot: Length of Meridians' states: 'Kidney *qi* reaches the ears. If kidney *qi* is in harmony, one can hear the five notes[①].' The elderly, with their declining kidney function, may experience gradual or complete loss of hearing, or other problems of the auditory sense, like tinnitus. Some people may hear the sound like roaring, buzzing, or the chirping of cicadas in their ears. To treat tinnitus, one should differentiate a deficiency pattern from an excess pattern.

Q3. What does it mean that the kidney opens to the two private parts?

The two private parts are called 'two *yin*' in TCM, that is, anterior *yin* and posterior *yin*, referring to the external genitalia and anus. Problems of urination and defecation are also frequently attributed to the kidney in TCM. Many elderly people suffer from dysuria, frequent micturition, and edema (particularly over the shin bone area). Others complain about constipation or loose bowels. One condition of the latter in TCM is called the fifth-watch diarrhea (early morning loose bowels), which compels patients to hurry to the restroom upon waking up at dawn each day. All these conditions have a lot to do with the kidney.

Q4. How does kidney *qi* impact urination and defecation?

According to *Huangdi's Inner Canon of Medicine*, the urinary bladder governs urination. 'The bladder is the reservoir officer, responsible for storing fluids. When *qi* is transformed, urine is excreted from the body,' according to 'Fundamental Questions: Secret Canon Stored in the Royal Library.' That the bladder is the reservoir officer means the bladder is the place where fluids are gathered. Fluids stored in the bladder cannot be excreted on their own. They have to be transformed into urine by the movement of *qi* for discharge.

The TCM bladder is different from the physical organ for urination. It is

---

① five notes: referring to the five musical notes that rise in pitch, from *gong* (宫 do), *shang* (商 re), *jue* (角 mi), *zhi* (徵 sol) to *yu* (羽 la).

exterior-interiorly related to the kidney in TCM. The kidney has the function of transforming the water in the bladder into fluids, with some transmitted to other parts of the body and some turned into urine. However, when kidney *qi*, that is, *yang qi*, is insufficient, this transformation process is deterred, thus causing difficulty in urinating. Children sometimes wet the bed, because their kidney *qi* is still growing, yet to mature. To sum up, when there is urine abnormality, a TCM physician would usually consider treatment from the kidney aspect.

Similarly, defecation is closely connected with the kidney. Deficient kidney *qi* results in difficulty in defecation. If deficient kidney *qi* is accompanied with heat, one tends to have dry and hard stool. If kidney *yang* is insufficient, one is likely to have loose bowels.

Some of the elderly have excessive internal heat, with dry mouth, a constant thirst for water, soreness in the lower back, weakness in the legs, lack of strength, and constipation. A possible TCM diagnosis would be 'kidney fire in a deficient condition flaming upward' and it should be treated by replenishing *yin* and purging fire. During the treatment, patients are recommended to consume food with the replenishing effects such as medlar, mulberry, walnut and so on while spicy food should be avoided.

If soreness in the lower back and lack of strength are accompanied by dizziness, it indicates a deficiency pattern. In this case, kidney deficiency should be tackled by tonifying the kidney *qi* instead of replenishing *yin*. A common prescription is River-water Facilitating Decoction (*Jì Chuān Jiān* 济川煎) whose chief herbs such as Desert-living Cistanche (*ròu cōng róng* 肉苁蓉) and Medicinal Cyathula Root (*chuān niú xī* 川牛膝) have the effect of tonifying kidney *qi* and boosting the patient's strength. During the treatment, patients should avoid exposure to cold weather and cold food, while food with a replenishing effect is recommended, for instance, mutton.

The fifth-watch diarrhea often occurs between 3 a.m. to 5 a.m., the time period when roosters crow and when the night shifts into day. TCM believes when one arises, one's inner *yang qi* escapes, resulting in a comparatively deficient state of inner *yang qi*, insufficient to arrest incontinence of stool. So, the mechanism of this pattern is in fact the insufficiency of kidney *yang*, also called kidney *yang* deficiency.

A TCM prescription named Four-miracle Pill (*Sì Shén Wán* 四神丸) is known for its effect of tonifying kidney *yang*, astringing the intestines, and arresting incontinence. It contains four medical herbs: Evodia Fruit (*wú zhū yú* 吴茱萸), Nutmeg (*ròu dòu kòu* 肉豆蔻), Chinese Magnoliavine Fruit (*wǔ wèi zǐ* 五味子), and Malaytea Scurfpea Fruit (*bǔ gǔ zhǐ* 补骨脂). Besides this, Chinese chives and mutton are also recommended to supplement kidney *yang*.

Q5. What is the relationship between the kidney and the bones?

The bones also have a close connection to the kidney. Since marrow is generated in the bones, it is also under its influence. Essence is transformed into marrow, and since essence is governed by the kidney, marrow can be seen as generated by the kidney. That is why TCM treatments of marrow diseases usually start with regulating the kidney. As 'Miraculous Pivot: The Seas in the Human Body' (*Líng Shū Hǎi Lùn* 灵枢•海论) states, 'the brain is the sea of marrow.' Hence, for brain diseases, treatment can also begin from the kidney aspect. For instance, tonifying the kidney helps to boost brain development, commonly used in the following conditions such as fontanelle problems, late talkers, brain paralysis, seizures and so on.

Children with attention deficit and hyperactivity disorder (ADHD) can also be treated by tonifying the kidney as the first step since the root cause is insufficient brain development. When insufficient brain development is accompanied by fire syndrome, often resulting in the pattern of fire harassing the mind and lack of concentration, treatment should focus on purging heart fire and removing phlegm-heat.

According to TCM, the kidney governs the bones that support the human body. Among toddlers, late walkers may indicate poor kidney *qi* development. Young adults may slip and fall without getting bone injuries because their kidney *qi* is in its prime, while the elderly people are more susceptible to bone fractures such as Colles fractures and femoral neck fractures, a consequence of insufficient kidney *qi*. With insufficient kidney *qi*, less marrow is generated. With insufficient marrow, the bones are not well-nurtured and thus rendered frail. Hence, for the elderly, kidney care should not be ignored.

Also governed by the kidney are the teeth, 'the extension of the bones.' Late dental growth in children and gomphiasis in the elderly are both obvious examples of the close connection between the two parts.

Q6. How does kidney *qi* impact hair?

Nowadays, women attach great importance to their hair care. In fact, the splendor of one's hair relies not on hair care products but on the wellness of the kidney. One's hair volume grows as one matures, along with the growth of one's kidney *qi*. In old age, hair starts falling and turning grey along with the decline of kidney *qi*. Therefore, replenishing one's kidney is a good therapy to nourish hair.

Young people with grey hair, however, cannot be all categorized as having kidney problems. It may have to do with mental stress, hyperactivity of liver fire and heat in blood. A case in point is the story of one's hair turning white overnight. There is a household story in China. Wu Zixu (伍子胥), a historical militarist in the late Spring and Autumn Period (770–476 BC) was hunted by King Ping of Chu and cast in a desperate situation. With two tall mountains and a river blocking his way and the only pass heavily fortified, he was overwhelmed by anxiety and his hair turned white overnight. Since it is too far-fetched to assume his kidney *qi* declined over just a few hours, his condition has more to do with intense stress and hyperactivity of heart fire and liver fire. Purging heart and liver fire and removing heat from blood are correct treatments in similar cases. In daily life, one can take in an appropriate amount of black sesame and walnut as food supplements to nourish hair.

Q7. What is the emotion most apt to affect the kidney?

Among the seven emotions of joy, anger, anxiety, overthinking, sorrow, fear, and fright, fear is the one apt to affect the kidney. If one is too overwhelmed by excessive fear or constantly in fear, diseases are prone to occur. 'Fundamental Questions: Pain' states: 'Excessive fear drives *qi* downward.' In colloquial language there is the expression 'be so scared as to wet one's pants.' Incontinence of urination is the consequence of *qi* sinking, which fails to arrest urine.

In TCM, fright (*jīng* 惊) and fear (*kǒng* 恐) are two separate emotions. They impair the kidney if in excess. Fright refers to the fact that unexpected external stimulants trigger palpitation and mental distraction giving rise to the disorder of *qi* flow. As is stated in 'Fundamental Questions: Pain,' 'when one is frightened, then the heart has nothing to lean on, the spirit has nowhere to return and one's deliberation has nowhere to settle.' Fear, on the contrary, is derived from within. Fear springs from one's inner heart, as one is usually afraid and worried that something one dreaded in the past might happen again. Fright and fear are frequently put together into one word—panic (*jing kong* 惊恐), referring to the state of one being frightened first and then being afraid. That is, when one is taken by surprise, one is easily scared. From the perspective of TCM, when one's kidney *qi* is insufficient, fright may linger and develop into fear.

'Fundamental Questions: Significant Discussions on Phenomena Corresponding to *Yin* and *Yang*' states that overthinking conquers fear. Overthinking pertains to earth, the spleen; while fear pertains to water, the kidney. To overcome fear, overthinking is the way. One relevant case records a lady struck by fear in the Jin dynasty (1115–1234). When she was staying at an inn one night, burglars broke in. She was so startled that she fell off the bed and passed out. After the incident she became so paranoid that she'd faint at any little unexpected noise. Even her maids had to tiptoe around the house to avoid startling her. The lady saw quite a few physicians with little improvement. All those who treated her proposed regulating her heart since emotional disorder is mostly related to the heart which governs spirit. But none of the therapies or prescriptions were effective. Eventually, her family turned to the renowned physician Zhang Congzheng (张从正) for help. Zhang proposed an innovative solution. He presented a tea table with a wood chip on it in front of the lady (with one maid at each of her sides) and asked her what she saw. 'A table and a wood chip,' she replied. Then the physician slapped the wood chip onto the tabletop right in front of her face, making a huge noise. She fainted immediately.

When she woke up, he comforted her, assuring her it was nothing but a wood chip and a table, with no harm at all. Then he slapped the chip repeatedly. In addition, he sent people to knock on the lady's window and door at night on purpose. Over time, the lady gradually got better and did not get startled easily. In fact, she recovered so completely that even thunder could not startle her, according to the original record of this case in *Confucians' Duties to Their Parents*.

'Fundamental Questions: Significant Discussions on the Most Important and Abstruse Theory' proposes a treatment method called '*jing zhe ping zhi*' (惊者平 之), which is generally interpreted as the one who is frightened should be calmed. Zhang Congzheng, nevertheless, had a different understanding of the word *ping* (平). He interpreted the text as normalizing the fright instead of calming it. That is, to help the patient understand fear and to assure the patient that the stimulant is indeed harmless. In modern psychological terms, his therapy is a typical example of systematic desensitization of behavior. In TCM, this is a classic case of relieving fear by overthinking.

Q8. What is the relationship between the kidney and water?

The kidney is intertwined with the concept of water. 'Fundamental Questions: Genuine *Qi* Endowed by Heaven in Remote Antiquity' states: 'The kidney controls water. It receives and stores essence from the five *zang*-organs and the six *fu*-organs. Thus, only when the five *zang*-organs and the six *fu*-organs are vigorous can the kidney have enough essence to discharge.' Here in this context, water can be understood as essence. In some other parts of *Huangdi's Inner Canon of Medicine*, water simply refers to literal water. For example, 'Fundamental Questions: Disharmony' states: 'The kidney is an organ of water and governs fluids.' Here 'water' refers to the fluids involved in human metabolism. The kidney pertains to *yin*, so does water. Those with the *yin* quality have the tendency to descend, so the kidney (water) is in the lower position of our torso. To transform water into fluids and transmit them to other parts of the human body, *yang qi* is required to steam the water, and the kidney is the major organ responsible for this function. Accordingly, problems with water metabolism, for instance, edema, can be attributed to the disorder of the kidney. Through replenishing and tonifying the kidney, one can facilitate its function to transform water into fluids that flow to other parts of the body. Hence, 'Fundamental Questions: Acupoints to Treat Water and Heat Diseases' (*Sù Wèn Shuǐ Rè Xuè Lùn* 素问·水热穴论) states that when the *qi* of the lower part rises, it associates with the steaming function of kidney *yang*.

If the water transformation process is interrupted, edema, abdominal dropsy or hydrothorax may occur, which indicates one's *yang qi* is insufficient to transform water (*yin*). Insufficient *yang qi* can be further categorized into two types respectively: *yang qi* deficiency and *yang qi* stagnancy. To treat the former, physicians should tonify *yang qi*. For the latter, activating *yang qi* or unblocking yang is more appropriate.

According to a famous physician named Ye Tianshi (叶天士) of the Qing dynasty, inducing diuresis rather than warming *yang* should be focused on to activate *yang qi*. Thus, a common way to remove the blockage of *yang qi* is to induce secretion of urine to remove stagnant water.

Q9. What is the relationship between the kidney and the winter season?

The kidney corresponds to winter, the coldest time of the year. 'Fundamental Questions: Important Ideas in the Golden Chamber' (*Sù Wèn Jīn Kuì Zhēn Yán Lùn* 素问·金匮真言论) states: 'The north wind arises in winter. It causes illness in the kidney.' In other words, the kidney is more dominant in health issues in the winter season. Clinically, many patients have seasonal conditions that can be interpreted by this connection. One female patient in her thirties reported she had cold and purple hands with pain. These symptoms occurred with the onset of winter at first but remained persistent regardless of the season for the following two years. Later, there was even an ulcer on one of her fingers. The time of the first onset of her disease implied the insufficiency of kidney *yang* in a cold environment. Eventually she was cured by medicinals which tonified her kidney *yang*.

The text elaborates on the connection between the kidney and the winter season as follows. 'Diseases caused by the *qi* of the winter always involve the four limbs' and '*bi jue* (痹厥, numbness and coldness of the four limbs) always occurs in winter.' The TCM term *bi jue* is formed by two characters, *bi* (痹) referring to blockage or impediment and *jue* (厥) referring to reverse cold. Some heart diseases in TCM are called '*xiong bi*' (胸痹, blockage in the chest), with major symptoms of stuffiness in the chest and shortness of breath. Others are more prone to asthma in winter. Tonifying the kidney is a good starting point to cure these diseases.

Chapter 17
Nourishing the Kidney Is Nourishing Life

Q1. Why is nourishing the kidney paramount to preserving health?

As indicated in the previous two chapters, the kidney is the root of prenatal constitution. It governs inheritance and is closely connected to the life process of a human being from birth to growth, maturity, senility, and to death. It is also closely related to the other parts of the human body, for instance, bones, marrow, lower back, teeth, hair, ears, and the two private parts. In a nutshell, the kidney is of pivotal importance to one's health, and hence is called the root of prenatal constitution or the innate foundation.

Huangdi's Inner Canon of Medicine, a work on health preservation, assigns paramount importance to the well-being and the nourishing of the kidney. Relevant principles and regimens on kidney care can be found in the following part.

Q2. What does health preservation mean?

In short, to preserve health or nurture life is to preserve life. More specifically, it is a healthcare activity that makes use of certain methods to promote health, prevent disease, and prolong life. For some people, health preservation is reduced to a narrow sense of living a long time. In the past, one of the titles that Chinese people used to refer to their emperor is the 'Lord of Ten Thousand Years,' wishing the emperor to live a long life. As can be seen, longevity has been a common goal for all of humanity, and immortality an ideal long sought after. However, not only the length of life but also its quality matters. Health preservation aims at cultivating an appropriate lifestyle that ensures a lasting and desirable living experience.

Q3. What are the general principles of health preservation?

Huangdi's Inner Canon of Medicine proposes principles for preserving health, stating in 'Fundamental Questions: Genuine *Qi* Endowed by Heaven in Remote Antiquity' that 'the sages in remote antiquity who knew the tenets for cultivating health followed the principles of *yin* and *yang* and regulated and nourished essential *qi* with *shu shu* (术数, literally techniques and numbers).' Two principles are highlighted here: 1) abiding by the rules of *yin* and *yang*; and 2) regulating and nourishing essential *qi* with *shu shu*. The former requires people to follow the law of nature and the rules of natural human growth and development. The latter asks people to coordinate various ways of cultivating health. *Shu shu* refers to the specific ways of cultivating health in terms of living habits and exercise. For whatever method, moderation is the key.

Q4. What are the principles of keeping the kidney healthy?

To improve the well-being of the kidney, one must also follow the two general principles. First and foremost, one needs to understand the two natural characteristics of the kidney and comply with them.

The first feature of the kidney is its preference for stillness.

It is clearly stated in 'Fundamental Questions: Six-Plus-Six System and the Manifestations of the Viscera' that 'the kidney, analogous to *zhe* (蛰), is the root of storage.' *Zhe* refers to dormant insects or animals, known for their stillness in winter. They hibernate throughout the winter season without eating, drinking, urinating or defecating until the Awakening of Insects[①] (*jīng zhé* 惊蛰) of the following year, which usually begins on March 5th or 6th and signals the coming of spring. As is stated in 'The Book of Rites: Monthly Ordinances' (*Lǐ Jì Yuè Lìng* 礼记•月令), 'the winds of winter will conclude' at that time of the year. Insects will be awakened by the spring thunder and start to move about.

The hibernating insects sleep all winter and do not eat, drink, or exercise at all. This penchant for inactivity is shared by the kidney. Hence, to preserve the kidney, you must avoid overstrain as is stated in 'Fundamental Questions: Genuine *Qi* Endowed by Heaven in Remote Antiquity.' Besides, one should also avoid eating too much spicy food as it may impair *yang qi* in the body. In a word, overwork or disturbance of *yang qi* goes against the principles of preserving kidney health.

The kidney is analogous to hibernating insects not only because the two share the same trait of stillness, but because they both harbor strong life force. The dormant insects, upon the arrival of spring thunder, wake up from their hibernation and start to hunt for food, exhibiting their vigorous life force. Likewise, despite its penchant for calmness, the kidney stores innate life force.

The second feature of the kidney is its role as 'the root of storage,' which is stated in 'Fundamental Questions: Six-Plus-Six System and the Manifestations of the Viscera.' In previous chapters I elaborated on the essence stored in the kidney. It contains innate essence inherited from parents and ancestors, and the essence of the five *zang*-organs and six *fu*-organs. For this role of storage, over-discharge should be avoided. Instead, to facilitate the protection of the essence and strengthen the kidney is a principle of health cultivation.

Winter is the season that corresponds to the kidney; hence it is the most effective time to nourish this organ of water. 'Fundamental Questions: Significant Discussions on Regulating the Spirit in Accordance with the *Qi* of the Four Seasons'

---

① Awakening of Insects: one of the 24 solar terms according to traditional Chinese lunar calendar.

states: 'The three months of winter are the season for closing and storing. The water freezes and the earth cracks open. Care must be taken not to disturb *yang qi*.' Specifically, the text continues, one should 'sleep early at night and rise late in the morning, waiting for the sun to shine; one should conceal thoughts and wishes as if one had secrets or as if one had obtained what was desired.' Of course, with the fast pace of life in modern society, it is almost impossible to go to bed at nightfall, but these texts offer a direction for cultivating health in winter. One is also reminded to keep emotions and thoughts within rather than revealing them to others.

Furthermore, 'Fundamental Questions: Significant Discussions on Regulating the Spirit in Accordance with the *Qi* of the Four Seasons' states: 'One should avoid the cold and keep warm. Do not allow sweating as it causes the loss of *yang qi*.' This again underscores the importance of protecting *yang qi* and avoiding over-discharge and disturbance. Perspiration only occurs when *yang qi* acts on *yin*. Along with sweat flowing out of the skin, *yang qi* is also lost. In terms of the ideal time for exercise, morning is a good time since *yang qi* in nature and in the human body are rising and vigorous. If possible, one should avoid exercise in the evening time. In addition, taking in nourishing and tonifying food, such as some Chinese herbal pastes and replenishing soups to supplement kidney *qi* or essence, is also recommended in winter. All these measures emphasize storage, the key to health preservation of the kidney in the winter season.

The second principle of preserving kidney health is to comply with the natural growth and development of the human body in accordance with age. As discussed in the previous chapters, the kidney is the basis of human growth. It is specially related to reproduction. In the first two stages of life, around the ages of between 7 and 14 for a female and 8 and 16 for a male, kidney *qi* is rising and growing. 'Miraculous Pivot: Natural Span of Life' states: 'At the age of ten years old, one's five *zang*-organs have developed and are permeated with blood and *qi*. With the *qi* in the lower part, one tends to run.' In the first two stages of life, children begin to develop their kidney *qi*. Tonifying at this period is unnecessary except if they present morbid conditions of hypoplasia.

In the following two stages of life when a woman reaches the age between 21 and 28 and a man between 24 and 32, kidney *qi* is vigorous and in its prime. Along with this abundance, one's muscles and *zang-fu* organs are mature. That is why young adults are rarely fatigued and tend to break their biological cycle, staying up late and eating irregularly. They may feel alright at the time, but problems may occur when they get older. So, do not over-consume energy. One should not go against routine to overexert oneself. Otherwise, one might invite harm to their body.

Next, when a woman is at the age of 35 or around 42, and a man at the age of 40 or around 48, health reaches its prime and starts declining. Just as 'Fundamental Questions: Significant Discussions on Phenomena Corresponding to *Yin* and *Yang*' puts it, 'when one reaches 40 years old, half of *yin qi* (referring to kidney *qi*) has already been consumed; early aging begins to appear in one's daily activities.' Therefore, self-discipline and restraint are even more crucial for health preservation in this stage. One should avoid burning the midnight oil. Excessive exercise should also be avoided. Some people in this age bracket are very keen on exercise and overstrain their body by swimming five times a week or hiking twice a week. Consequently, their joints or organs suffer, and health is affected. In fact, moderate exercise like walking or strolling is more suitable for middle-aged people. Brisk walking in particular is an effective and accessible way to promote health.

Certain nourishing food and prescriptions with kidney-tonifying effects are also recommended for people in this age group. A famous case documented in an ancient medical work is about an old gentleman with a pitch-black beard and hair at the age of 80. His secret of healthcare was taking the Six-ingredient Rehmannia Pill and Pulse-activating Drink (*Shēng Mài Yǐn* 生脉饮) from the age of 40 onward. That means he had started tonifying the kidney since his middle age. According to *Commentaries on Ancient and Modern Case Records* (*Gǔ Jīn Yī Ǎn Àn* 古今医案按), taking Six-ingredient Rehmannia Pill in combination with Pulse-activating Drink throughout the year can regulate and cultivate health by addressing the root cause. Usually when one is over 40 years old, one's health is on the decline. Past 50, one starts to step into old age, with *qi* at the state of insufficiency in multiple organs including the kidney and the heart. The root cause of this inevitable decline is the insufficiency of kidney *qi*. Elderly people with chronic diseases might have kidney *qi* impaired even if their primary diseases have nothing to do with the kidney. This indicates that the kidney is the decisive factor of one's physical strength. That is why by supplementing kidney *qi*, one can slow down the aging process. Common herbal supplements include the above-mentioned two prescriptions. Besides, American Ginseng (*xī yáng shēn* 西洋参), Sanchi (*sān qī* 三七), and Chinese Caterpillar Fungus (*dōng chóng xià cǎo* 冬虫夏草) are also good for delaying aging. One can grind the three ingredients into powder and mix them in the ratio of 1:1:1 and take them on a regular basis.

In conclusion, health preservation of the kidney should be in line with the season, with the two characteristics of the kidney, and with the age of people. Physicians can facilitate the growth of the kidney, for teens, secure its well-being for the middle aged and tonify it for the elderly if necessary.

Q5. How do you preserve kidney health?

Here are a few specific ways to nurture the kidney in your daily life.

First, take herbal and food supplements.

Herbal and food nurturing are most frequently used. However, you must first make sure which kidney-deficiency pattern is the case in question. There are mainly three types: kidney *qi* deficiency, kidney *yin* deficiency, and kidney *yang* deficiency.

Kidney *qi* deficiency is characterized by lower back pain, weakness in the legs, lack of strength, and early aging symptoms such as amnesia, insomnia, hearing loss, hair loss or grey hair, and tooth loss. One recommended food for this pattern is Chinese Yam, which can be taken as food and used as a medicinal herb. Mild-natured with no toxicity, Chinese Yam can be a long-term medication. Its sweet flavor indicates its effect of invigorating the spleen and tonifying the lung as well as the kidney. It can be added into daily cuisine in multiple ways, for instance, stewed, steamed, or stir-fried. One medicinal cuisine-cum-dessert, Chinese Yam, and Goji Berry Congee, includes Chinese Yam and Goji Berry as the main ingredients. The congee can be sweetened with rock sugar and boiled down to a thick and sticky mixture, served as a dessert to tonify kidney *qi*. Furthermore, Chinese Yam also acts as one of the chief herbs in some well-known TCM prescriptions such as the Six-ingredient Rehmannia Pill and Golden-chamber Kidney *Qi* Pill (*Jīn Kuì Shèn Qì*

Wán 金匮肾气丸).

People with kidney *yin* deficiency demonstrate similar symptoms of kidney *qi* deficiency including lumbar aching, weakness in the legs, and lack of strength, but with some additional symptoms such as vexation, irritability, heat sensation in the palms, soles, and chest, dizziness, tinnitus, dreamfulness, insomnia, night sweating, tidal fever and so on. One medicinal herb-cum-food particularly suitable for this pattern is Goji Berry. Sweet in flavor and mild in property, it enters the kidney and the liver meridians, great for nourishing kidney *yin*. One can cook some delicious congee with Non-glutinous Rice, Goji Berry, and Black Sesame to tonify the kidney.

Goji Berry enjoys great popularity amongst people keen on health preservation. The ancient Chinese people glorified this herb, extolling its magical anti-aging effect. This is exemplified in a legend documented in Ishinpo (*Yī Xīn Fāng* 医心方) compiled by a Japanese scholar named Tamba Yasuyori in the year of 984. An official on a business trip in today's Sichuan province saw a young woman hitting a silver-haired old man by a river. Outraged by this, the official stopped her and demanded: 'How could you bully an old man?' The young woman answered: 'This is my great-grandson I was beating.' Shocked, the official asked how old she was. 'I am over 300 years old,' she replied. 'My grandson is only just over 80. I instructed him to take the Herb of Immortality, but he didn't listen. That's why he became so old. I was disciplining him for this.' Upon inquiry, the official was told that the Herb of Immortality was Goji Berry. The way she used this herb was somewhat different from how people use it in modern times. Nowadays people only use the berries, but the woman made use of most parts of the goji tree including its root, stem, leaf, and seed, and collected them at different times of the year. She employed different processing methods for different parts and consumed them throughout the year. This was her secret recipe for youth and longevity. The legend might not be true, but it does give an insight into how Chinese ancestors valued this medicinal herb and its anti-aging effect. One should bear in mind that Goji Berry is a tonic herb for replenishing the kidney.

Finally, kidney *yang* deficiency is characterized by symptoms such as lumbar aching, weak legs, aversion to cold, cold hands and feet as well as spontaneous sweating. Some might experience constipation or loose stools. In such cases, patent medicine like Golden-chamber Kidney *Qi* Pill can be used. Medicinal herbs such as Songaria Cynomorium Herb (*suǒ yáng* 锁阳) and Eucommia Bark (*dù zhòng* 杜仲) are also suitable, and foods with similar effects are recommended, including mutton and prawns. All these are warm in nature and are aimed to tonify kidney *yang*.

To sum up, nourishing the kidney is the key to health preservation in winter. The herbal treatments and food supplements mentioned above should be determined regarding their indications. Inappropriate treatments could result in counterproductive side-effects. Those with kidney *qi* insufficiency can take Six-ingredient Rehmannia Pill and Golden-chamber Kidney *Qi* Pill and eat Chinese Yam and Goji Berry Congee; those with kidney *yin* insufficiency can eat Black Sesame and Goji Berry Congee; and those with kidney *yang* insufficiency can take Golden-chamber Kidney *Qi* Pill and eat mutton, prawns and so on to boost *yang qi*.

Second, massage *yong quan* (涌泉 KI 1) acupoint.

The next way to improve kidney health is massaging *yong quan*, an acupoint of the kidney meridian, located near the anterior 1/3 of the sole. This point is right in the anterior depression when the foot is flexed. (See Figure 17-1)

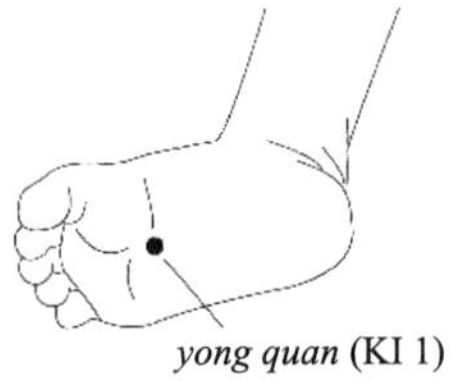

yong quan (KI 1)

Figure 17-1　*Yong quan* acupoint

There are three ways to massage the point. The first is to push it in the direction of the toes, the second is to knead it, and the third is to rub it with warm palms. That is, rub your palms together until they feel warm before you rub the point in a circular motion.

Massaging *yong quan* acupoint has a good effect on nourishing and tonifying the kidney. It can be dated back to the Song dynasty (960–1279) when it was already a popular regimen among civilians. The great literary figure of the Northern Song dynasty, Su Dongpo (苏东坡) documented an anecdote in his works on health pre-servation. South China (the area that comprises the present-day Fujian province and

Guangdong province) was frequently plagued by pestilent *qi* at the time. While many fell ill, one military officer managed to remain healthy and radiant though in a highly contaminable environment. His secret was that every morning when he got up, he sat with his soles pressed against each other and massaged *yong quan* acupoint with his hands until he started to sweat. Others quickly followed suit and fended off the epidemic. This therapy was handed down through the passage of time.

The currently popular foot bath, in fact, is also one way of massaging *yong quan* acupoint. For people who take foot baths, remember to keep the water temperature up and add warm water frequently. Water in the tub should be high enough to soak the ankles. Since one perspires easily when taking foot bath, one should also remember to drink water to avoid dehydration. For the old and frail as well as diabetes patients, foot baths are not recommended.

Third, swallow saliva.

A third way to nurture the kidney is swallowing saliva. According to 'Fundamental Questions: Elucidation of Five *Qi*,' 'the fluids are transformed from the five *zang*-organs... the kidney generates spittle.' The kidney collateral extends to *lian quan* (廉泉 CV 23) acupoint at the root of the tongue where spittle comes out. TCM believes spittle, the thin saliva, is transformed from the essence in the kidney and should not be spat out. Instead, it should be swallowed to nourish the kidney.

The method can be found in 'Fundamental Questions: Needling Methods'[①] (*Sù Wèn Cì Fǎ Lùn* 素问•刺法论). Those with chronic kidney disease should face south at *yin shi* (寅时, 3 to 5 a.m.), tranquilizing the mind and eliminating avarice, holding their breath (only inhalation and no exhalation) seven times, stretching their neck to take a deep breath like swallowing something hard seven times. Then, saliva underneath the tongue is swallowed. It should be performed between 3 and 5 a.m. because the period from early morning to noon is *yang* of *yang*.

In daily life, you can simplify the procedure by clicking your teeth to produce more saliva. Click teeth 36 times to 72 times in the morning, and then swirl your tongue clockwise and anticlockwise, each for 9 times to 18 times. When you feel saliva build up in your mouth, puff out your cheeks a couple of times to produce even

---

① 'Fundamental Questions: Needling Methods': Some believe that the original version was lost and this one was supplemented in the Northern Song dynasty (960–1127).

more. Then slowly swallow the saliva down three times, with the mind picturing it descending all the way down to *dan tian* (丹田, lower elixir field) which is 3 *cun* (寸) or approximately 10 cm below the navel. Incidentally, girls nowadays love to wear crop tops that expose the navel, around which there are three acupoints: *shen que* (神阙 CV 8), *qi hai* (气海 CV 6), and *guan yuan* (关元 CV 4). All are points where kidney *qi* is infused. This may result in coldness around the belly where kidney *qi* is located and cause painful periods, irregular menstruation, and even difficulty in conceiving a baby. It is more than necessary to repeatedly highlight the importance of keeping the lower abdomen warm to protect kidney *qi*. (See Figure 17-2)

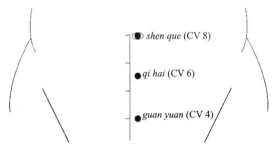

Figure 17-2　Acupoints around the navel

As you now know, swallowing saliva is one of the ways recorded in *Huangdi's Inner Canon of Medicine* to help people nourish the kidney. Today, it has become one of the *qigong* methods to strengthen the body. Besides this, clicking teeth has also grown into a way of health preservation, as teeth are believed to be the extension of the bones which are governed by the kidney.

In conclusion, several ways have been introduced to help you strengthen the kidney, including having adequate potent herbs, eating nutritive congee, massaging *yong quan* acupoint, and swallowing saliva. Remember that the kidney is the innate foundation of the body, thus it can be said that nourishing the kidney is nourishing life.

Appendix I
Ancient Books

Titles in Chinese *Pinyin*	Titles in Chinese	Titles in English
Bái Shì Nèi Jīng	《白氏内经》	Master Bai's Inner Classic
Bái Shì Wài Jīng	《白氏外经》	Master Bai's Outer Classic
Běn Cǎo Cóng Xīn	《本草从新》	Newly Revised Materia Medica
Běn Cǎo Gāng Mù	《本草纲目》	Compendium of Materia Medica
Biǎn Què Nèi Jīng	《扁鹊内经》	Bianque's Inner Classic
Biǎn Què Wài Jīng	《扁鹊外经》	Bianque's Outer Classic
Chóng Guǎng Bǔ Zhù Huáng Dì Nèi Jīng Sù Wèn	《重广补注黄帝内经素问》	Huangdi's Inner Classic Fundamental Questions: Broadly Corrected and Re-annotated
Chūn Qiū Fán Lù	《春秋繁露》	Luxuriant Gems of the Spring and Autumn Annals
Dào Zàng	《道藏》	Collected Daoist Scriptures
Ěr Yǎ	《尔雅》	Er Ya
Fù Qīng Zhǔ Nǚ Kē	《傅青主女科》	Fu Qingzhu's Obstetrics and Gynecology
Gǔ Jīn Yī Àn Àn	《古今医案按》	Commentaries on Ancient and Modern Case Records
Guǎn Zǐ	《管子》	Guanzi
Guǎng Yùn	《广韵》	Various Rhymes
Hán Fēi Zǐ	《韩非子》	Hanfeizi

Hán Shì Yī Tōng	《韩氏医通》	*Han's General Medicine*
Hàn Shū	《汉书》	*The History of the Han Dynasty*
Huái Nán Zǐ	《淮南子》	*Huainanzi*
Huáng Dì Bā Shí Yī Nàn Jīng	《黄帝八十一难经》	*Huangdi's Eighty-one Difficult Issues*
Huáng Dì Míng Táng Jīng	《黄帝明堂经》	*Huangdi's Brightness Hall Classic*
Huáng Dì Nèi Jīng	《黄帝内经》	*Huangdi's Inner Canon of Medicine*
Huáng Dì Wài Jīng	《黄帝外经》	*Huangdi's Outer Canon of Medicine*
Jiǔ Juàn	《九卷》	*Nine Volumes*
Lán Shì Mì Cáng	《兰室秘藏》	*Secrets from the Orchid Chamber*
Lèi Jīng	《类经》	*Classified Classics*
Liè Zǐ	《列子》	*Liezi*
Líng Shū	《灵枢》	*Miraculous Pivot*
Lǚ Shì Chūn Qiū	《吕氏春秋》	*Master Lü's Spring and Autumn Annals*
Míng Táng Wǔ Zàng Lùn	《明堂五脏论》	*Brightness Hall Discourse on the Five Zang-Organs*
Míng Yī Lèi Àn	《名医类案》	*Classified Medical Records of Distinguished Physicians*
Nàn Jīng	《难经》	*Classic of Difficult Issues*
Páng Piān	《旁篇》	*Appended Chapters*
Pí Wèi Lùn	《脾胃论》	*Treatise on the Spleen and Stomach*
Qī Lüè	《七略》	*Seven Summaries*
Qiān Jīn Fāng	《千金方》	*Prescriptions Worth a Thousand Pieces of Gold*
Rú Mén Shì Qīn	《儒门事亲》	*Confucians' Duties to Their Parents*
Rú Lín Wài Shǐ	《儒林外史》	*The History of Confucian School*
Sān Guó Yǎn Yì	《三国演义》	*The Romance of the Three Kingdoms*
Sān Guó Zhì	《三国志》	*Records of the Three Kingdoms*
Shāng Hán Lùn	《伤寒论》	*Treatise on Cold Damage*

Shāng Hán Zá Bìng Lùn	《伤寒杂病论》	*Treatise on Cold-damage and Miscellaneous Diseases*
Shàng Shū	《尚书》	*The Book of History*
Shén Nóng Běn Cǎo Jīng	《神农本草经》	*Shennong's Herbal*
Shén Shū	《神枢》	*Spirit Pivot*
Shǐ Jì	《史记》	*Records of the Historian*
Shuǐ Hǔ Zhuàn	《水浒传》	*Water Margin*
Shuō Wén Jiě Zì	《说文解字》	*Explanation of Scripts and Elucidation of Characters*
Sù Wèn	《素问》	*Fundamental Questions*
Xiǎo Ér Yào Zhèng Zhí Jué	《小儿药证直诀》	*Key to Diagnosis and Treatment of Children's Diseases*
Yì Jīng	《易经》	*I Ching/Book of Changes*
Yī Xīn Fāng	《医心方》	*Ishinpo*
Yī Xué Rù Mén	《医学入门》	*Introduction to Medicine*
Yù Shū	《玉枢》	*Jade Pivot*
Zhēn Jīng	《针经》	*Classic of Acupuncture*
Zhēn Jiǔ Jiǎ Yǐ Jīng	《针灸甲乙经》	*Classic of Acupuncture in the Systematic Classic of Acupuncture and Moxibustion*
Zhōng Guó Yī Jí Kǎo	《中国医籍考》	*Textual Research on Chinese Medical Classics*
Zhōng Guó Zhé Xué	《中国哲学》	*History of Chinese Philosophy*
Zhōu Shèn Zhāi Yī Xué Quán Shū	《周慎斋医学全书》	*Complete Medical Works by Zhou Shenzhai*
Zhuāng Zǐ	《庄子》	*Zhuangzi*

Appendix II
Some Chapters in *Huangdi's Inner Canon of Medicine*

Titles in Chinese *Pinyin*	Titles in Chinese	Titles in English
Líng Shū Bǎi Bìng Shǐ Shēng	灵枢·百病始生	Miraculous Pivot: The Occurrence of All Diseases
Líng Shū Běn Shén	灵枢·本神	Miraculous Pivot: Basic State of Spirit
Líng Shū Běn Shū	灵枢·本输	Miraculous Pivot: Acupoints
Líng Shū Běn Zàng	灵枢·本脏	Miraculous Pivot: The Viscera as the Foundation of Human Beings
Líng Shū Cháng Wèi	灵枢·肠胃	Miraculous Pivot: Intestines and the Stomach
Líng Shū Dà Huò Lùn	灵枢·大惑论	Miraculous Pivot: Great Perplexity
Líng Shū Hǎi Lùn	灵枢·海论	Miraculous Pivot: The Seas in the Human Body
Líng Shū Jīng Mài	灵枢·经脉	Miraculous Pivot: Meridians
Líng Shū Jīng Shuǐ	灵枢·经水	Miraculous Pivot: The Relationship Between Rivers and Channels
Líng Shū Jiǔ Zhēn Lùn	灵枢·九针论	Miraculous Pivot: Nine Needles
Líng Shū Jiǔ Zhēn Shí Èr Yuán	灵枢·九针十二原	Miraculous Pivot: Nine Needles and Twelve Origins

Líng Shū Jué Qì	灵枢•决气	Miraculous Pivot: Differentiation of *Qi*
Líng Shū Kǒu Wèn	灵枢•口问	Miraculous Pivot: Questions and Answers
Líng Shū Lùn Yǒng	灵枢•论勇	Miraculous Pivot: Bravery
Líng Shū Mài Dù	灵枢•脉度	Miraculous Pivot: Length of Meridians
Líng Shū Píng Rén Jué Gǔ	灵枢•平人绝谷	Miraculous Pivot: Fasting in Healthy People
Líng Shū Tiān Nián	灵枢•天年	Miraculous Pivot: Natural Span of Life
Líng Shū Wǔ Wèi	灵枢•五味	Miraculous Pivot: Five Flavors
Líng Shū Xié Kè	灵枢•邪客	Miraculous Pivot: Pathogenic Invasion
Líng Shū Yíng Wèi Shēng Huì	灵枢•营卫生会	Miraculous Pivot: Generation and Convergence of Nutrient *Qi* and Defense *Qi*
Líng Shū: Xié Qì Zàng Fǔ Bìng Xíng	灵枢•邪气脏腑病形	Miraculous Pivot: Symptoms of *Zang-Fu* Organs due to the Invasion of Pathogenic *Qi*
Sù Wèn Bǎo Mìng Quán Xíng Lùn	素问•宝命全形论	Fundamental Questions: Treasuring Life and Preserving Physical Appearance
Sù Wèn Bì Lùn	素问•痹论	Fundamental Questions: *Bi*-syndrome
Sù Wèn Bìng Tài Lùn	素问•病能论	Fundamental Questions: Manifestations of Diseases
Sù Wèn Cì Fǎ Lùn	素问•刺法论	Fundamental Questions: Needling Methods
Sù Wèn Cì Jìn Lùn	素问•刺禁论	Fundamental Questions: Contraindication of Needling Therapy
Sù Wèn Fēng Lùn	素问•风论	Fundamental Questions: Wind

Sù Wèn Fù Zhōng Lùn	素问·腹中论	Fundamental Questions: Abdominal Diseases
Sù Wèn Jīn Guì Zhēn Yán Lùn	素问·金匮真言论	Fundamental Questions: Important Ideas in the Golden Chamber
Sù Wèn Jīng Mài Bié Lùn	素问·经脉别论	Fundamental Questions: Special Discussion on Meridians and Vessels
Sù Wèn Jǔ Tòng Lùn	素问·举痛论	Fundamental Questions: Pain
Sù Wèn Ké Lùn	素问·咳论	Fundamental Questions: Cough
Sù Wèn Líng Lán Mì Diǎn Lùn	素问·灵兰秘典论	Fundamental Questions: Secret Canon Stored in the Royal Library
Sù Wèn Liù Jié Zàng Xiàng Lùn	素问·六节藏象论	Fundamental Questions: Six-Plus-Six System and the Manifestations of the Viscera
Sù Wèn Liù Wēi Zhǐ Dà Lùn	素问·六微旨大论	Fundamental Questions: Significant Discussions on the Abstruseness of the Six Kinds of *Qi*
Sù Wèn Liù Yuán Zhèng Jì Dà Lùn	素问·六元正纪大论	Fundamental Questions: Significant Discussions on the Changing Principles of Six *Qi*
Sù Wèn Mài Yào Jīng Wēi Lùn	素问·脉要精微论	Fundamental Questions: Essentials of Pulse Taking and the Subtleties of Pulse Manifestation
Sù Wèn Nì Tiáo Lùn	素问·逆调论	Fundamental Questions: Disharmony
Sù Wèn Píng Rén Qì Xiàng Lùn	素问·平人气象论	Fundamental Questions: Pulse Conditions of Healthy People
Sù Wèn Qí Bìng Lùn	素问·奇病论	Fundamental Questions: Strange Diseases
Sù Wèn Rè Lùn	素问·热论	Fundamental Questions: Heat
Sù Wèn Shàng Gǔ Tiān Zhēn Lùn	素问·上古天真论	Fundamental Questions: Genuine *Qi* Endowed by Heaven in Remote Antiquity

Sù Wèn Shēng Qì Tōng Tiān Lùn	素问·生气通天论	Fundamental Questions: The Interrelationship Between Life and Nature
Sù Wèn Shuǐ Rè Xuè Lùn	素问·水热穴论	Fundamental Questions: Acupoints to Treat Water and Heat Diseases
Sù Wèn Sì Qì Tiáo Shén Dà Lùn	素问·四气调神大论	Fundamental Questions: Significant Discussions on Regulating the Spirit in Accordance with the *Qi* of the Four Seasons
Sù Wèn Tài Yīn Yáng Míng Lùn	素问·太阴阳明论	Fundamental Questions: Greater *Yin* and *Yang* Brightness
Sù Wèn Tāng Yè Láo Lǐ Lùn	素问·汤液醪醴论	Fundamental Questions: Soups and Liquors
Sù Wèn Tiān Yuán Jì Dà Lùn	素问·天元纪大论	Fundamental Questions: Significant Discussions on the Law of Motions and Changes of Original *Qi* in the Universe
Sù Wèn Wěi Lùn	素问·痿论	Fundamental Questions: Flaccidity
Sù Wèn Wǔ Cháng Zhèng Dà Lùn	素问·五常政大论	Fundamental Questions: Significant Discussions on the Administration of Five Motions
Sù Wèn Wǔ Zàng Shēng Chéng Piān	素问·五脏生成篇	Fundamental Questions: Various Relationships of the Five *Zang*-Organs
Sù Wèn Xuān Míng Wǔ Qì Piān	素问·宣明五气篇	Fundamental Questions: Elucidation of Five *Qi*
Sù Wèn Yí Jīng Biàn Qì Lùn	素问·移精变气论	Fundamental Questions: Change of Essence and Transformation of *Qi*
Sù Wèn Yīn Yáng Yìng Xiàng Dà Lùn	素问·阴阳应象大论	Fundamental Questions: Significant Discussions on Phenomena Corresponding to *Yin* and *Yang*
Sù Wèn Yù Jī Zhēn Zàng Lùn	素问·玉机真脏论	Fundamental Questions: Genuine-*zang* Pulses

Sù Wèn Zàng Qì Fǎ Shí Lùn	素问·藏气法时论	Fundamental Questions: *Qi* in the *Zang*-Organs Following the Rules of Seasonal Changes
Sù Wèn Zhì Zhēn Yào Dà Lùn	素问·至真要大论	Fundamental Questions: Significant Discussions on the Most Important and Abstruse Theory

Appendix Ⅲ
Chinese Medicinals

Names in Chinese *Pinyin*	Names in Chinese	Names in English
ài yè	艾叶	Argy Wormwood Leaf
bái sháo	白芍	White Peony Root
bái tóu wēng	白头翁	Chinese Pulsatilla Root
bái zhǐ	白芷	Dahurian Angelica Root
bái zhú	白术	White Atractylodes Rhizome
bàn xià	半夏	Pinellia Tuber
bò he	薄荷	Peppermint
bǔ gǔ zhǐ	补骨脂	Malaytea Scurfpea Fruit
cāng ěr zǐ	苍耳子	Siberian Cocklebur Fruit
chái hú	柴胡	Chinese Thorowax Root
chán yī	蝉衣	Cicada Slough
chén pí	陈皮	Dried Tangerine Peel
chì sháo	赤芍	Red Peony Root
chuān liàn zǐ	川楝子	Szechwan Chinaberry Fruit
chuān mù tōng	川木通	Armand Clematis Stem
chuān niú xī	川牛膝	Medicinal Cyathula Root
cí shí	磁石	Magnetite
dà huáng	大黄	Rhubarb
dān pí	丹皮	Tree Peony Bark
dān shēn	丹参	Danshen Root

dāng guī	当归	Chinese Angelica
dǎng shēn	党参	Tangshen
dōng chóng xià cǎo	冬虫夏草	Chinese Caterpillar Fungus
dù zhòng	杜仲	Eucommia Bark
fáng fēng	防风	Divaricate Saposhnikovia Root
fú líng	茯苓	Poria Cocos
gān cǎo	甘草	Licorice Root
gān cǎo shāo	甘草梢	Tip of Licorice Root
gě gēn	葛根	Kudzuvine Root
gǒu qǐ zǐ	枸杞子	Barbary Wolfberry Fruit/Goji Berry
guā lóu	瓜蒌	Snakegourd Fruit
guì zhī	桂枝	Cassia Twig
huáng lián	黄连	Golden Thread
huáng qí	黄芪	Milkvetch Root
huáng qín	黄芩	Baical Skullcap Root
huò xiāng	藿香	Agastache
jiāng cán	僵蚕	Stiff Silkorm
jié gěng	桔梗	Platycodon Root
jīng mǐ	粳米	Non-glutinous Rice
lú rú/qiàn cǎo	蘆茹 / 茜草	Indian Madder Root
mài dōng	麦冬	Dwarf Lilyturf Root
máng xiāo	芒硝	Sodium Sulfate
pèi lán	佩兰	Fortune Eupatorium Herb
piàn jiāng huáng	片姜黄	Wenyujin Concise Rhizome
qián hú	前胡	Hogfennel Root
qín pí	秦皮	Ash Bark
rén shēn	人参	Ginseng
ròu cōng róng	肉苁蓉	Desert-living Cistanche
ròu dòu kòu	肉豆蔻	Nutmeg
ròu guì	肉桂	Cassia Bark
sān qī	三七	Sanchi
shā shēn	沙参	Adenophora Root

shān yào	山药	Common Yam Rhizome/Chinese Yam
shān zhū yú	山茱萸	Asiatic Cornelian Cherry Fruit
shēng dì	生地	Unprocessed Rehmannia Root
shēng jiāng	生姜	Fresh Ginger
shēng lóng gǔ	生龙骨	Raw Dragon Bone
shēng mǔ lì	生牡蛎	Raw Oyster Shell
shēng shí gāo	生石膏	Raw Gypsum
shú dì	熟地	Prepared Rehmannia Root
shú mǐ	秫米	Broomcorn Millet
sū yè	苏叶	Perilla Leaf
suān zǎo rén	酸枣仁	Spine Date Seed
suǒ yáng	锁阳	Songaria Cynomorium Herb
tiān dōng	天冬	Asparagus Root
wáng bù liú xíng	王不留行	Cow-herb Seed
wǔ wèi zǐ	五味子	Chinese Magnoliavine Fruit
wū zéi gǔ/hǎi piāo xiāo	乌贼骨/海螵蛸	Cuttlefish Bone
wú zhū yú	吴茱萸	Evodia Fruit
xī yáng shēn	西洋参	American Ginseng
xiè bái	薤白	Longstamen Onion
xīn yí	辛夷	Biond Magnolia Flower
xìng rén	杏仁	Apricot Seed
yù jīn	郁金	Turmeric Root Tuber
zé xiè	泽泻	Water-plantain Rhizome
zhī mǔ	知母	Common Anemarrhena Rhizome
zhǐ shí	枳实	Immature Orange Fruit
zhī zǐ	栀子	Cape-Jasmine Fruit
zhú rú	竹茹	Bamboo Shavings
zhú yè	竹叶	Lophatherum Herb

Appendix IV
Traditional Chinese Medicine Formulas

Names in Chinese *Pinyin*	Names in Chinese	Names in English
Bā Zhèng Sǎn	八正散	Eight-ingredient Ratification Powder
Bái Hǔ Tāng	白虎汤	White Tiger Decoction
Bàn Xià Shú Mǐ Tāng	半夏秫米汤	Pinellia Tuber and Broomcorn Millet Decoction
Bǔ Zhōng Yì Qì Tāng	补中益气汤	Center-tonifying *Qi*-replenishing Decoction
Chái Qín Wēn Dǎn Tāng	柴芩温胆汤	Bupleurum and Scutellaria Gallbladder-warming Decoction
Dà Chéng Qì Tāng	大承气汤	Major Purgative Decoction
Dāng Guī Bǔ Xuè Tāng	当归补血汤	Angelica Decoction for Tonifying Blood
Dǎo Chì Sǎn	导赤散	Redness-removing Powder
Guā Lóu Xiè Bái Bái Jiǔ Tāng	瓜蒌薤白白酒汤	Decoction of Snakegourd Fruit, Longstamen Onion and *Bai Jiu*
Guì Zhī Gān Cǎo Tāng	桂枝甘草汤	Cassia Twig and Licorice Decoction
Guì Zhī Tāng	桂枝汤	Cinnamon Twig Decoction
Huáng Lián Ē Jiāo Tāng	黄连阿胶汤	Golden Thread and Donkey-hide Glue Decoction

Jì Chuān Jiān	济川煎	River-water Facilitating Decoction
Jiāo Tài Wán	交泰丸	*Jiao Tai* Pill
Jīn Guì Shèn Qì Wán	金匮肾气丸	Golden-chamber Kidney *Qi* Pill
Lán Cǎo Tāng	兰草汤	Decoction of Fortune Eupatorium Herb
Pái Dú Yǎng Yán Jiāo Náng	排毒养颜胶囊	Detox and Beauty Capsule
Qì Zhì Wèi Tòng Kē Lì	气滞胃痛颗粒	Granules for *Qi*-stagnation Stoma-chache
Shēng Jiàng Sǎn	升降散	Ascending and Descending Powder
Shēng Mài Yǐn	生脉饮	Pulse-activating Drink
Sì Shén Wán	四神丸	Four-miracle Pill
Wū Zéi Gǔ Lǘ Rú Wán	乌贼骨蘆茹丸	Cuttlefish Bone and Indian Madder Root Pill
Xiāo Yáo Sǎn	逍遥散	Carefree Powder
Xiè Huáng Sǎn	泻黄散	Spleen-Purging Powder
Yáng Gān Wán	羊肝丸	*Yang Gan* Pill
Yù Píng Fēng Sǎn	玉屏风散	Jade Wind-Barrier Powder
Yuè Bì Tāng	越婢汤	Maidservant from Yue Decoction
Zǎo Rén Ān Shén Yè	枣仁安神液	Spine Date Seed Drink for Calming Spirit
Zhū Fū Tāng	猪肤汤	Pig Skin Decoction

Appendix V
Chronology of Chinese History*

Five Emperors (Huangdi, Zhuanxu, Diku, Yao, and Shun)		early 3000 BC–early 2100 BC
Xia dynasty		2070 BC–1600 BC
Shang dynasty		1600 BC–1046 BC
Western Zhou dynasty		1046 BC–771 BC
Eastern Zhou dynasty	Spring and Autumn Period	770 BC–476 BC
	Warring States Period	475 BC–221 BC (Zhou fell in 256 BC)
Qin dynasty		221 BC–206 BC
Han dynasty	Western Han dynasty	206 BC–AD 25
	Eastern Han dynasty	25–220
Three Kingdoms	Wei	220–265
	Shu	221–263
	Wu	222–280
Jin dynasty	Western Jin dynasty	265–317
	Eastern Jin dynasty	317–420

(to be continued)

Southern and Northern dynasties	Southern dynasties	Song	420–479
		Qi	479–502
		Liang	502–557
		Chen	557–589
	Northern dynasties	Northern Wei	386–534
		Eastern Wei	534–550
		Northern Qi	550–577
		Western Wei	535–556
		Northern Zhou	557–581
Sui dynasty			581–618
Tang dynasty			618–907
Five dynasties		Later Liang	907–923
		Later Tang	923–936
		Later Jin	936–947
		Later Han	947–950
		Later Zhou	951–960
Song dynasty		Northern Song dynasty	960–1127
		Southern Song dynasty	1127–1279
Liao dynasty			907–1125
Jin dynasty			1115–1234
Yuan dynasty			1206–1368
Ming dynasty			1368–1644
Qing dynasty			1616–1911
Republic of China			1912–1949
The People's Republic of China			Founded on October 1, 1949

* Cited from *Key Concepts in Chinese Thought and Culture I*, Foreign Language Teaching and Research Press, 2015: 141–142.